Clinical Methods and Practicum in Audiology

Singular Textbook Series
Series Editor: M. N. Hegde, Ph.D.

Child Phonology: A Book of Exercises for Students
by Ken Bleile, Ph.D.

Clinical Methods and Practicum in Speech-Language Pathology
by M. N. Hegde, Ph.D., and Deborah Davis, M.A.

Applied Phonetics: The Sounds of American English
by Harold T. Edwards, Ph.D.

Applied Phonetics Workbook: A Systematic Approach to Phonetic Transcription
by Harold T. Edwards, Ph.D., and Alvin L. Gregg, Ph.D.

Teacher's Manual for Applied Phonetics
by Harold T. Edwards, Ph.D.

Clinical Methods and Practicum in Audiology
by Ben R. Kelly, Ph.D., Deborah Davis, M.A., and M. N. Hegde, Ph.D.

Also Available

A Singular Manual of Textbook Preparation
by M. N. Hegde

Consulting Editor
Jeffrey Danhauer, Ph.D.
Professor, University of California at Santa Barbara

Clinical Methods and Practicum in Audiology

Ben R. Kelly, Ph.D.
Deborah Davis, M.A.
M. N. Hegde, Ph.D.

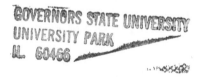

SINGULAR PUBLISHING GROUP, INC.
San Diego, California

Singular Publishing Group, Inc.
4284 41st Street
San Diego, California 92105-1197

® 1994 by Singular Publishing Group, Inc.

Typeset in 10½/12 Garamond by House Graphics
Printed in the United States of America by BookCrafters

Library of Congress Cataloging-in-Publication Data
Kelly, Ben Reily, 1942-
    Clinical methods and practicum in audiology / Ben R. Kelly,
Deborah Davis, M. N. Hegde.
        p.   cm. — (Singular textbook series)
    Includes bibliographical references and index.
    ISBN 1-56593-161-0
    1. Audiology—Study and teaching (Internship) 2. Audiology—
Practice.   I. Davis, Deborah, 1951- . II. Hegde, M. N.
(Mahabalagiri N.), 1941- . III. Title. IV. Series.
RF291.K45   1993
617.8—dc20
                                                                    93-28364
                                                                        CIP

Contents

v

Appendixes

Index / 345

Preface

Students finish their preclinic requirements and look forward to the next stage in their training with mixed feelings. They feel excited about having progressed to this point. They experience anxiety about working with actual clients. Students are unsure of the requirements of clinical practicum. After all, practicum means applying their skills and knowledge. Yet, their preparation so far has been academic and theoretical. It is little consolation to students entering clinical practicum that instructors and clinical supervisors have judged them ready. To complicate matters further, many students mistakenly feel that instruction, and with it room for error, is behind them. They are relieved to find that clinical practicum has room for learning and, therefore, room for error. For students who are enrolling in practicum for the first time, it is important to know the structure of the experience and what organizational, professional, and ethical rules are to be followed in service delivery.

This book is for students entering practicum in audiology. However, it is not written solely for audiology majors. We realize that speech-language pathologists take audiology practicum and have attempted to keep them in mind as we addressed the areas of audiology practicum they are most likely to experience.

Students sense a gap between their academic preparation and clinical practicum. They have heard other students talk about practicum; about administrative differences among practicum sites; about difficult clients, writing reports, staffings, and other activities they may not have experienced. Much of the art and many of the skills needed for a successful practicum experience are not discussed in the textbooks or in class. This text was written to fill the gap between academic preparation and clinical practicum. It is intended as a text or reference book for clinical practicum. However, those who read it before enrolling in practicum may approach the experience with less apprehension.

The book is organized into four parts. Part I provides insight into the structure and function of clinical practicum. In it, we have given an overview of the experience, discussed preclinic requirements, specified ASHA guidelines related to practicum, and explained students' responsibilities and supervisors' expectations.

Parts II through IV provide insight into the delivery of services. Part II deals with the planning and delivery of effective hearing conservation programs and how to organize, conduct, and evaluate audiologic services efforts in various settings. Part III gives a strategy for approaching diagnostics. Part IV presents a strategy for approaching the management of clients with communicative difficulties resulting from hearing loss. Students are expected to have the course work to support their delivery of services. They are informed at intervals what background is expected of them, and, in general, where in their academic course work specific material is usually covered. Background material that is readily available in textbooks is not repeated. For example, we saw little need to describe the standard procedure for accomplishing the pure-tone audiogram. However, specific procedures for service delivery are outlined when they are not readily available in textbooks. Each procedure presented is listed in the table of contents under the appropriate chapter heading for easy reference by the student.

We wrote all parts of the text from a practical orientation. We have emphasized that practicum is a learning experience. We cite few references. We present little research. We discuss few theories. References, substantiating research, and theoretical discussion are handled in academic textbooks. We present ways of delivering service, ways that emphasize the art of service delivery, as well as the science. This book emphasizes that clinical practicum facilitates the student in becoming a competent clinician.

We realize that this book presents some very specific information. We believe that different programs deliver quality service through a variety of organizational frameworks. Many individual supervisors have unique individual approaches to practicum. We believe that variety in the methods of accomplishing quality clinical practicum experience is a strength in our profession. We can only hope that this book is a source of information that clinical supervisors and student clinicians can build on and from which they can expand. We welcome input from clinical supervisors and students who may wish to share unique procedures and experiences that may be included in future revisions of this book.

We wish to acknowledge Dr. Stephen D. Roberts of Valley Children's Hospital in Fresno, California for reading the manuscript at its various stages and for his many valuable suggestions. We must also acknowledge our families, without whose support this project could not have been completed.

Part I

Clinical Practicum

Y ou will begin your clinical practicum after you have completed certain courses in audiology. Although you will have acquired some basic knowledge about hearing and its disorders, you will not have had any practical experience in audiological assessment and rehabilitation. Therefore, Part I includes information on the organization of audiologic clinical practicum, the conduct of the student clinician, interaction between the clinical supervisor and the student clinician, and general principles of working with clients. It is designed to give you an overview of practicum in audiology and thus help you prepare for it. You must read this part very carefully because much of this information may not have been offered to you in your academic courses.

Parts II, III, and IV include information on clinical methods used in the practice of audiology, reviewing the procedures most frequently used in hearing conservation and in the identification and management of clients with hearing disorders.

1

Clinical Practicum in Audiology

A udiology is the study of normal and disordered hearing. It is both a scientific discipline and a clinical profession. As a scientific discipline, audiology is concerned with normal hearing and its physical, psychological, behavioral, and social bases. As a clinical profession, it is concerned with assessment and management of hearing impairment in children and adults. Therefore, as a student in audiology, you are required to obtain both academic knowledge through course work and practical experience through supervised clinical work. You learn about normal and disordered hearing, assessment of hearing, and management of persons with hearing impairment through academic course work. Through clinical practicum, you acquire professional skills in assessing hearing loss by using standardized procedures, interpreting the results, and planning and implementing management or rehabilitation programs for persons with hearing problems. Therefore, training programs in audiology reflect the dual concerns of scientific knowledge and professional skills.

Your training in audiology begins with academic course work necessary to acquire background knowledge. The academic portion of the training program emphasizes theoretical and scientific information. In various courses, you will learn about hearing, speech, and language, and communication. Although some of the academic courses must be taken before you begin your clinical practicum, others may be taken concurrently.

After you have completed prerequisite academic courses, you may be ready for practical training offered through clinical practicum. The clinical practicum gives you an opportunity to learn the skills of a professional audiologist with the help of a clinical supervisor. This dual training at the academic and practical levels provides you with the technical knowledge and clinical skills to practice the profession of audiology.

An Overview

Audiological clinical practicum is a supervised experience in which you learn professional skills of assessing and managing people with hearing disorders. It is designed to prepare you for your future role as a professional audiologist. Participation in clinical practicum allows you to use and integrate the information obtained in your academic course work. All audiology programs accredited by the American-Speech-Language-Hearing Association (ASHA) require you to enroll in clinical practicum.

Some undergraduate students begin clinical practicum in their senior year. Most students, however, begin their practicum during the first semester of graduate study. A few students may take part in limited clinical practice in their junior year. In this case, the undergraduate student may observe and assist other student clinicians providing clinical services. As the student learns some of the basic skills, greater participation may be allowed. The student initially may assist in preparing audiological equipment before the session and take notes during the client interview. Eventually, the student may begin to administer pure-tone screenings or evaluations as the primary clinician.

At some universities, the first clinical experience for audiology majors is their practicum in speech-language pathology. Because audiology and speech-language pathology are closely related professions, students in both areas are required to complete a minimum level of clinical practicum in the other area. To fulfill the speech-language pathology practicum that ASHA requires of audiology majors, student clinicians evaluate and manage clients with speech or language disorders. Some students question the utility of practicum in an area in which they will not be certified. However, practicum in speech-language pathology is extremely useful for audiologists. Hearing impairment in children may be associated with speech and language problems. Even adults with hearing impairments may have speech and language difficulties. Therefore, many clients seen by audiologists need speech-language pathology services. With practicum in speech-language pathology, audiology students gain a better understanding of all individuals, including those with hearing difficulties who exhibit speech or language disorders. Therefore, practicum in speech-language pathology will help future audiologists in counseling their clients and making appropriate referrals for speech-language pathology services. Likewise, many clients seen by speech-language pathologists need audiological services. With practicum in audiology, speech-language pathology students gain a better understanding of the needs of individuals with hearing disorders. Such an understanding will help future speech-language pathologists in counseling their clients and making appropriate referrals for audiologic services.

Supervisors try to assign less complex cases to beginning student clinicians. Supervisors also consider whether students have had relevant courses before assigning clients. For example, beginning graduate students in audiology take courses in the fundamentals of audiological evaluation and management. In clinical practicum, these students may administer basic test batteries and be involved in some counseling of individuals with hearing losses. Audiology majors also may have completed all the requisite courses to complete their practicum in speech-language pathology and be assigned one or two clients with a speech or language disorder. During subsequent semesters, audiology majors enroll in more advanced audiology course work including courses on differential diagnostic procedures and hearing aid analysis. The students then will be assigned the clients with more complex disorders. They may work with clients who need extensive testing, including advanced auditory brainstem response testing, electronystagmography, or central auditory processing evaluations. They also will be more involved in counseling clients with hearing loss and in selecting, fitting, and dispensing hearing aids.

In most training programs, speech-language pathology students taking audiology practicum are able to meet requirements within a single registration. Even though speech-language pathologists may have completed one or more semesters of practicum in speech-language pathology, they are still beginning student clinicians in audiology practicum. Therefore, they are assigned audiologic cases only after they have had introductory courses in audiology.

The American Speech-Language-Hearing Association (ASHA) requires that speech-language pathology students get a mix of basic diagnostic and management experiences in audiology practicum. Therefore, speech-language pathology students are assigned less complex audiologic cases. For example, speech-language pathology students may count the time they spend screening hearing of schoolchildren for their diagnostic hours. The students also may complete a portion of their management hours managing speech and language disorders in children with hearing impairments. A positive note for the speech-language pathology students with one or more semesters of practicum in speech-language pathology is that their experiences in dealing with clients transfer to audiology practicum, enabling them to complete the audiology practicum without the stress of a first-time clinical experience.

University clinics are not always able to assign clients based on academic experience. Some universities provide student clinicians with a variety of clients each term. For example, a first semester graduate student may not have had a class in hearing aids. However, because of the expertise of the clinical supervisor, the student may be assigned a client who needs hearing aids. The supervisor provides the amount of instruction and supervision the student requires to serve the client effectively and appropriately.

Clinical practicum assignments will involve both on- and off-campus clinical sites. Most universities require student clinicians to complete a minimum number of clinical hours at the on-campus clinic before they are assigned to off-campus practicum sites. Initially, students provide audiology services at the university clinic under the supervision of a university supervisor. Later, an audiologist from the university, from the off-campus facility, or both may supervise audiology practicum. Clinical practicum assignments may include hospitals, schools, community hearing centers, private practices, physicians' offices, or various other clinical sites.

As you progress in your clinical and academic program, you will be given more responsibility in planning, evaluating, and managing clients. You will not be expected to work independently or know everything as a beginning student clinician. Your clinical supervisor will help you prepare for sessions and research necessary information. As your clinical experience increases, you will be required to perform more independently in most of your clinical responsibilities. Although you will be supervised throughout all your student practica, you eventually will be expected to provide effective clinical service with little input from your supervisor.

General Preclinic Requirements

Several skills will contribute to your success in clinical practicum. Of course, it is important that you acquire solid academic knowledge. However, in addition to a strong academic foundation, you need to develop many other skills, including good written and oral communication skills which are described in this section. You should work toward acquiring some of these skills before you begin your clinical practicum.

There also are less tangible personal characteristics without which you cannot successfully complete your clinical practicum. For example, you must be able to plan and organize your time efficiently. Equally important will be your ability to perform reliably and responsibly. However, no supervisor expects you to have all the necessary skills at the beginning of your first semester of clinical practicum. You will be expected to learn from your experiences and interactions with your supervisor.

Academic Requirements

You will complete preclinic academic requirements both at the undergraduate and graduate levels. Along with students in speech-language pathology, you probably will take undergraduate courses on phonetics, anatomy and physiology of the speech and hearing mechanisms, acoustics, speech science, articulation and phonology, and the development of language in children. Courses in introductory audiometry also are often taken at the undergraduate level. You may take courses in speech and language disorders as preparation for your participation in speech-language pathology practicum. A course in aural rehabilitation also may be offered at the undergraduate or graduate level.

In graduate courses, you obtain more advanced information on all aspects of hearing disorders, their assessment, and management. Being technical and research-based, the graduate courses build on the information offered at the undergraduate level and emphasize specialized information. For example, besides taking advanced courses in principles of audiology, you also take courses such as instrumentation, pediatric audiology, industrial audiology, hearing aid analysis, electrical response audiology, and psychoacoustics.

Course requirements and sequences vary from university to university. However, as a general rule, students are expected to have completed introductory courses in normal and abnormal speech, language, and hearing development before beginning clinical practicum. They also should have completed introductory courses in speech and hearing sciences and audiometry. Your advisor will inform you about these and other requirements in the department. You should plan ahead for your clinical practicum by discussing the specific requirements with your advisor.

General Writing Requirements

Professional audiologists must write many reports in a short period of time. Therefore, professional practice requires good writing skills. To teach these skills, student clinicians are required to write numerous diagnostic reports, management summaries, and progress notes. In many audiology clinics, you may be required to write reports daily. These reports may be sent to clients, physicians, educational agencies, or other referral sources.

Before enrolling in clinical practicum, you are not expected to know all the technical terms or the specific formats used in writing these reports, but you should develop your general writing skills prior to beginning clinical practicum. You should learn to write clearly and concisely. You probably have taken several English classes in which you completed "creative" writing assignments using lengthy, descriptive, and complex sentences. In clinical report writing you communicate technical information, and you must write short, easily understood sentences. You must organize your thoughts coherently and avoid the use of ambiguous phrases. Of course, you must be able to write grammatically correct sentences that are free from spelling errors.

Some universities require student clinicians to use word processing programs in writing their reports. Compared to typing reports, a word processing package can make report writing much quicker and easier. As you write your first few reports, you can store them in the computer as templates or standard formats. Later you can copy the format and standard information and adapt the report for new clients.

Many word processing programs contain grammar and spelling checkers. If they do not, you can usually add spelling and grammar checkers to them. These programs will help you write more accurately, clearly, and simply.

You should discuss any concerns you have about your writing skills with your advisor as early in your program as possible. Your advisor may determine that your writing skills meet the preclinical writing requirements. If your writing skills need to be improved, your advisor may suggest a writing course or give you special writing assignments to complete. Practice in writing is essential. Contingent feedback on the quality of your writing and revision in light of the feedback also are essential. Becoming an efficient, effective writer will enhance your academic career and simplify your clinical practicum challenges.

Oral Communication Skills

Audiologists interact daily with people of all ages and from all walks of life. As a student audiologist, you will communicate not only with your clients and clinical supervisors, but also with a variety of other professionals including physicians, hearing aid manufacturers and distributors, speech-language pathologists, educators of the deaf, and other audiologists. You will develop some of the necessary communication skills in courses dealing with counseling and in clinical practicum.

Oral communication skills such as speaking clearly and succinctly should be developed before beginning clinical practicum. You should know when to use technical terms, when to simplify them, and when to substitute nontechnical terms. You should learn to speak in ways that facilitate comprehension by persons with hearing impairment. For example, you should speak slowly and only when your face is clearly visible to the person with hearing impairment.

Personal Characteristics

Besides technical knowledge and good written and oral communication skills, student clinicians are expected to have certain personal characteristics necessary for successful clinical practice. Responsible behavior is one important characteristic.

Student clinicians must take full responsibility for their professional actions. Therefore, you should be fully prepared for all clinical sessions. You should be highly responsible in your interactions with clients, their family members, clinical staff members, and your clinical supervisors. You should meet all deadlines. You should promptly schedule the clients that are assigned to you. Your diagnostic or assessment reports, management plans, progress notes, filling out various clinical forms, filing papers in the client folders, and so forth must be completed on time. You may have clinic appointments the same day a major report is due or a test is given in a class. Nonetheless, you must always be prepared in advance for each clinical session and attend each session for which you are scheduled.

An appropriate sense of humor is also an important asset for student clinicians to develop. Unusual and sometimes humorous situations often occur when working with people. Student clinicians should be able to recognize when the use of humor is acceptable. It is never acceptable to laugh at others or their misfortune. It is also not acceptable to laugh at racial, ethnic, or sexual slurs. However, it is certainly acceptable, and often helps a client feel more comfortable, to laugh with clients who see humor in their situations.

Because you are entering a helping profession, you should be able to empathize with your clients' problems and personal situations. You should combine your technical skills with a caring disposition. You should not regard your clients as scores on a test, but as individuals who happen to have certain difficulties. You should try to place your assessment results in the context of a person's living conditions and circumstances. For example, it is more meaningful to discuss not only the audiometric results, but also what the hearing handicap means to an individual and how it affects his or her personal, social, and occupational life.

As a student clinician, you should show systematic progress in working independently. Of course, your level of experience will determine how independent you can be in making clinical decisions. In your beginning practicum experiences, you most likely will depend on your supervisor to guide you through the clinical process. Even so, you still must be prepared to research clinical literature independently to find appropriate methods of practice. Your academic background should help you find technical information in books, journals, and other sources. If you are not familiar with advanced diagnostic instruments and equipment, you should spend extra time in advance of scheduled appointments to learn how to use them. Your supervisor will help you learn how to evaluate the efficacy and accuracy of your clinical sessions, determine areas of needed change, and make appropriate modifications that you or your supervisor identify.

The more clinical experience and academic knowledge you gain, the more independently you will be expected to perform. As a beginning student audiologist, your clinical supervisor might model administration of a new test, but as a more advanced student audiologist, your clinical supervisor may expect you to read and apply the test manual information without modeling. During your final clinical practicum, you should exhibit independent planning and judgment although you will still be under supervision. Student clinicians' responsibilities are discussed in more detail in Chapter 4.

Knowledge of the Profession and Related Agencies

Several accrediting, licensing, and professional organizations and government agencies affect your training and career as an audiologist. As you begin your training, you should have at least a basic knowledge of these organizations and agencies and the regulations related to the profession of audiology. The national professional organization that affects your training and professional career the most is the American-Speech-Language-Hearing Association (ASHA). If your state has a licensure law, the licensing agencies of your state for audiology and hearing aid dispensing also affect your profession.

The American Speech-Language-Hearing Association

ASHA is a national scientific and professional organization concerned with the professions of communicative disorders and the services people with those disorders receive. As you probably know, ASHA regulations play a significant role in shaping the twin disciplines of audiology and speech-language pathology as well as their training programs. Student clinicians will hear repeated references to ASHA and ASHA's requirements regarding clinical practicum. Your clinical practicum assignments and clinical supervision are greatly influenced by ASHA's requirements.

As an organization that acts as an advocate for individuals with communicative disorders and the professionals who provide services to these individuals, ASHA (ASHA Membership, 1991) has five primary goals:

1. To maintain high standards of clinical competence for professionals providing speech-language pathology and audiology services to the public.
2. To encourage the development of comprehensive clinical service programs.
3. To promote investigation of clinical procedures used in treating disorders of communication.

4. To stimulate exchange of information about human communication through conventions, publications, and other continuing professional education activities.
5. To encourage basic research and scientific study of human communication and its disorders. (p. 5)

ASHA addresses its goal of maintaining high standards of clinical competence in various ways. In addition to sponsoring conferences and workshops to encourage continuing professional education, ASHA offers an Award for Continuing Education. ASHA also collects and disseminates data related to research, clinical service delivery, education, and career opportunities. Over the years, ASHA has created several manuals, video and audio tapes, brochures, and other materials its members can purchase to help them enhance their service delivery.

ASHA has established accreditation and certification procedures that outline minimum standards of education and clinical service delivery. These standards are outlined in the form of academic and clinical preparation and include compliance with the ASHA Code of Ethics. University training programs that meet ASHA standards may receive **accreditation** from ASHA. ASHA accreditation should not be confused with accreditation of the university or college as a whole. ASHA accreditation is awarded to individual departments providing training in the area of audiology or speech-language pathology. Certain regional agencies may accredit entire universities or colleges. **Certification** is awarded to individuals who complete a program of study and clinical experience approved by ASHA. ASHA certification is known as the **Certificate of Clinical Competence** and more commonly referred to as the **CCC** or **Cs** (sees). This certificate may be in audiology, speech-language pathology, or both. Certification by ASHA in both audiology and speech-language pathology is referred to as **dual certification**. Remember, accreditation is awarded to programs, while certification is awarded to individuals.

Two of ASHA's agencies accredit academic programs and clinical services. The **Educational Standards Board (ESB)** accredits academic programs, and the **Professional Services Board (PSB)** accredits clinical services. A university has several options in seeking ASHA accreditation. It may request accreditation of its academic program, its clinical services, or both. Also, the university may seek accreditation for its speech-language pathology program, audiology program, or both. When applying for accreditation, the university submits a completed application form and documentation of its compliance with ASHA regulations. ASHA reviews the application and schedules a site visit with the university. ASHA usually sends one team of experts to evaluate the educational programs and another team to evaluate the clinical services offered by the university. If the university is applying for both ESB and PSB certification, ASHA will send one team to evaluate both programs. Only graduate degree programs are accredited by ASHA.

The ESB accreditation team evaluates the quality and number of faculty teaching courses, the curriculum offered by the department, the library and other resources of the university, and many other factors that affect the education of future speech-language pathologists and audiologists. The PSB accreditation team evaluates clinical services offered by the department. The team reviews the qualifications and certification status of clinical supervisors, adequacy of physical facilities and clinical equipment, and all other factors that affect the quality of clinical services offered to the public. Both teams also may schedule meetings to talk with current students as well as graduates of the program. After the site visits, each team submits a report to the ASHA Board they are responsible for (ESB or PSB). Based on these reports, the ESB and the PSB make a final decision on whether to accredit the program.

ASHA's stringent ESB and PSB requirements directly influence both you and your training program. First, if you are attending a program accredited by ASHA, you are assured that the department has minimally met ASHA's standards, guaranteeing you a good education. Second, graduates of ASHA ESB-accredited programs escape some of the cumbersome paperwork involved in applying for the Clinical Fellowship Year and Certificate of Clinical Competence. Third, beginning January 1, 1994, individuals must have graduated from an ESB-accredited program to be eligible for the Certificate of Clinical Competence.

As you now know, ASHA awards the Certificate of Clinical Competence (CCC) to individuals who have successfully met ASHA's academic, clinical, and ethical standards in speech-language pathology, audiology, or both. To be eligible for certification in audiology, you must satisfy the following requirements:

1. **Earn a Master's (M.A.) or Doctoral (Ph.D. or Au.D.) degree.** Because you will be applying for certification January 1, 1993 or later, you must hold a master's or doctoral degree in audiology. Prior to January 1, 1993, individuals applying for certification had to have held a master's degree or its equivalent. Equivalent course work without a master's degree no longer satisfies the minimum requirement for certification (ASHA Clinical Certification Board, 1992).

2. **Complete a Clinical Fellowship Year.** After you have completed the educational and clinical requirements at the college level, you are required to complete an internship, known as the Clinical

Fellowship Year (CFY). Although the CFY is an extension of your training as a professional, it may not be part of your university's training program. The CFY is designed to help you move effectively from the role of student clinician to professional. The CFY can be a paid or volunteer experience. Your work is supervised by a professional holding current ASHA certification in the same area in which you are seeking certification (speech-language pathology or audiology). The CFY can be completed in 9 months of full-time work (at least 30 hours per week), in 15 months of part-time work (20-24 hours per week, or in 18 months of part-time work (15-19 hours per week). Your CFY must be completed within 36 months from the date you initiate it. Note that the CFY must be completed within 7 years after you have finished your academic and practicum requirements. (ASHA Clinical Certification Board, 1992).

3. **Obtain a passing score on the National Examination in Speech-Language Pathology and Audiology (NESPA).** The NESPA is a comprehensive assessment of your knowledge in audiology. The examination consists of objective questions. The NESPA usually can be taken through your university's testing office. Many students find it best to take the NESPA as soon as they complete the academic portion of their training or soon after completing graduate comprehensive examinations.

4. **Know and adhere to the ASHA Code of Ethics.** You will become familiar with ASHA's Code of Ethics. You must be knowledgeable of changes in the code of ethics and comply with its various guidelines. Chapter 3 contains a more detailed discussion of the code of ethics.

5. **Submit your application for certification and pay your membership fee.** ASHA publishes a **Membership and Certification Handbook** which contains application forms as well as detailed information regarding academic, practicum, CFY, and membership requirements. You can contact ASHA to obtain this handbook. The current address and telephone number for ASHA are available in the journal, *Asha*. Individuals at the national office are also available to answer any questions you have regarding certification procedures.

The CCC does not imply any legal status. However, many state licensure requirements are based on the CCC requirements. The CCC is recognized as the minimum proficiency level for practice in most employment settings.

State Licensure Board for Audiology

States began licensing the practice of audiology in the late 1960s. In states that have a licensure law, ASHA's CCC is not always sufficient to practice audiology. Where you live and in what setting you practice determine whether you need to meet state licensure requirements. Whereas the CCC indicates you have met ASHA's minimum competency levels, licensure suggests you have met the minimum legal requirements for practice in your state.

A state board or committee for Audiology and Speech-Language Pathology will regulate **licensure** of audiologists and speech-language pathologists. Most states in the United States now have licensure requirements for audiologists. With the exception of a few states, the state licensure requirements are compatible with those of CCC. Many states also have licensure reciprocity with the CCC (Lynch, 1990). Some work settings may be exempt from licensure requirements. Audiologists who provide services in the public schools or federal government agencies commonly are exempt from licensure regulations.

State Licensure for Hearing Aid Dispensing

Since the mid-1970s audiologists have dispensed hearing aids in the management of individuals with hearing loss. In many states, dispensing hearing aids was a licensed activity prior to the licensure of audiology. As a result, audiologists who dispense hearing aids are required to obtain dispensing licenses. A state board or committee will regulate licensure of hearing aid dispensers. Audiologists working in federal government agencies and in some state agencies who dispense but do not sell hearing aids are often exempt from state laws regulating the dispensing of hearing aids.

American Academy of Audiology

The American Academy of Audiology (AAA) is an organization, established in 1988, whose primary mission is to improve "services to hearing-impaired individuals by advancing the highest professional standards of Audiology." Hood (1992) enumerated six goals that accompany the mission of the Academy:

1. Improve the evaluation and treatment of the hearing-impaired;
2. Promote public awareness of auditory disorders and hearing impairment;
3. Provide leadership in the formulation and upgrading of professional standards;
4. Disseminate the results of both basic and applied research through scholarly publications;

5. Disseminate information to the general public on current trends and developments in the profession; and

6. Provide a professional home for all audiologists. (p. 2)

The Academy promotes a professional doctorate as an entry level degree for the profession. Since its inception, AAA has shown remarkable growth. By June 1992 its membership had grown to 4,300 (Hood, 1992). All full-time graduate students enrolled in ESB-accredited audiology programs are eligible for complimentary subscriptions to the *Journal of the Academy of Audiology* and the bulletin, *Audiology Today*. Your program coordinator receives requests to update lists of graduate students periodically. Audiology graduate students probably will receive these publications automatically. However, if you do not and are eligible, simply request a letter verifying your status and mail it to AAA. The current address and telephone for AAA may be found in the *Journal of the American Academy of Audiology* or in *Audiology Today*.

Academy of Dispensing Audiology

The Academy of Dispensing Audiologists (ADA) is an organization whose primary goal is to represent the interests of audiologists who dispense and the hearing aid using public. They support the doctorate of Audiology (Au.D.) degree as the entry level degree for audiologists. The current address of the Academy of Dispensing Audiologists may be found in the *Journal of the Academy of Dispensing Audiologists*.

American Auditory Society

The American Auditory Society (AAS) is a scientific and research-oriented group open to all persons with interests in hearing and hearing loss. Its membership is composed of audiologists, physicians, hearing aid dispensers and manufacturers, educators of the deaf, and others.

The AAS provides complimentary copies of its journal, *Ear and Hearing*, to students in graduate audiology training programs. The current address and telephone number are: American Auditory Society, Inc., 1966 Inwood Road, Dallas, Texas 75235 [Telephone: (214) 330-4203].

Academy of Rehabilitative Audiology

"The purpose of the Academy of Rehabilitative Audiology (ARA) is to provide a forum for the exchange of ideas on, knowledge of, and experience with habilitative and rehabilitative aspects of audiology and to foster and stimulate professional education, research, and interest in habilitative and rehabilitative programs for hearing impaired persons" (ARA, 1992, p. 1). This organization supports the doctorate as the entry level degree for the practice of audiology. The address of this professional association changes as the officers of the association change. Your audiology supervisor may be able to provide you with the current address should you wish to affiliate with this organization as a student member.

State Departments of Education

State Departments of Education oversee public school employees. Student audiologists planning to work in the public schools often must obtain an educational credential or certificate issued by the state's department of education. Educational and practicum requirements for most educational credentials are similar to those of CCC and state licensure. However, requirements for the educational credential vary across states. For example, in addition to completing regular clinical practicum, you may be required to complete a practicum assignment in the public schools. A different requirement may be a certain number of hours required with children. Additional courses related to public school education or child development also may be required. Credential requirements are unique to individual states. Be sure to discuss your career plans with your advisor so you can fulfill all necessary requirements.

The National Student Speech-Language-Hearing Association

The National Student Speech-Language-Hearing Association (NSSLHA) is a student organization designed to involve students enrolled in speech-language pathology and audiology in their future professions. Local NSSLHA chapters are run by students with the help of faculty advisors. NSSLHA is affiliated with ASHA and is an excellent source of professional information.

NSSLHA chapters organize fund-raising activities, social events, and professional workshops and seminars. NSSLHA provides a forum for you and your fellow students to meet and discuss training and professional issues.

In addition to providing you with current professional information, membership in NSSLHA can help support you in your educational program by providing you discounts to professional publications, organizations, and events. NSSLHA membership dues are a fraction of the ASHA dues, yet you receive many of the same benefits offered to full dues paying professional members of ASHA. You will be able to attend the annual ASHA conference at a reduced rate and may be able to receive reduced rates for certain state conferences. Members of NSSLHA also receive ASHA journals. These journals are a valuable source of scientific and professional information you cannot do without. As a graduate student, you frequently will be asked to read journal articles, and you will appreciate the convenience of having your own journals. NSSLHA also publishes its own journal, *National Student Speech Language Hearing Association Journal,* which is distributed to its members.

Just as important, NSSLHA gives students the opportunity to begin developing a social and professional network with individuals who have similar interests. Early in your undergraduate program, become a member of the local chapter of NSSLHA. This membership will help you meet students with similar interests and assist you in keeping current on all aspects of your future profession.

ASHA Guidelines on Practicum

ASHA has designed broad, but comprehensive clinical practicum requirements. These requirements ensure that students receive thorough clinical training program. Students demonstrate that they have met the clinical practicum and internship requirements by satisfactorily completing clinical clock hours under the supervision of ASHA-certified speech-language pathologists or audiologists. ASHA mandates requirements for both students and supervisors. The following section emphasizes the requirements for students.

Clinical Observation

Your introduction to clinical practicum is through observation. You begin preparation for clinical practicum by observing the work of more experienced clinicians. In your observations, you will see how the information you have learned in academic courses is applied in the clinic, and you will begin to understand the assessment and management processes.

ASHA has established several guidelines for clinical observation. To meet the clinical observation requirements ASHA mandates students to do the following (ASHA Clinical Certification Board, 1992):

1. **Obtain a minimum of 25 clock hours of supervised clinical observation before beginning clinical practicum.** To broaden your clinical background and expand your knowledge, you may want to observe more than the minimum 25 clock hours. As you advance through your clinical program, you will find that you always learn from observing other clinicians.

2. **Observe live clinical sessions, videotaped sessions, or sessions on closed-circuit television.** Although you probably will observe mostly live clinical sessions, ASHA allows observation of videotaped sessions or live sessions on closed-circuit television monitors. Your training program will direct your observation schedule.

3. **Observe a variety of sessions.** You may observe both management and evaluation sessions. Observations may be of children or adults. Your 25 observation hours may include a combination of audiology and speech-language pathology observation. Your university may require a certain distribution of hours based on your professional area of emphasis. For example, as an audiology major, your department may require you to obtain the majority of your observation hours in the audiology clinic. In addition to observing a variety of clients, it is also important to observe some clients over a period of time to note the progression of services. You may first observe a client during the hearing evaluation, later during the hearing aid evaluation and fitting, and finally for the hearing aid follow-up appointment.

4. **Obtain observation hours under the supervision of individuals who are currently certified by ASHA.** The clinical supervisor must hold a current CCC in the area in which the observation hours are being obtained. You may observe professionals or student clinicians. Regardless of whom you observe, your observation hours must be supervised by individuals holding current ASHA certification.

Observation of Clinical Sessions

There are several components to each clinical session. The arrangement of the room and nonverbal communication of the clinician are examples of two variables that might influence service delivery. During your clinical observations you will learn to evaluate different aspects of each session critically. If possible, review the client's file or discuss the session with the clinician prior to observing. Your university will describe any record keeping or observation reporting requirements that you will need to complete. Your supervisor will help you observe the following:

1. Room arrangement
2. Seating arrangement in the audiology booth
3. How the clinician greets the client
4. How the clinician conducts the session:
   a. Diagnostic and management procedures
   b. Sensitivity to client needs.
5. How the clinician conducts the closing interview with the client
6. How the clinician terminates the session and dismisses the client.

Responsibilities of Student Observers

Student observers are guests in the clinical session. Regardless of how unobtrusive you try to be, when a new person is in the room, the clinic session tends to be slightly disrupted. Therefore, it is important for you to demonstrate responsible and conscientious behavior. It is equally important for you to exhibit ethical behavior. When observing at both on- and off-campus sites, comply with the following guidelines:

1. **Schedule observations according to the clinic's guidelines.** There is little excess space in the audiological suite. To avoid being crowded or denied access to the clinical session, schedule your observation appointments in advance.

2. **Arrive on time for observations.** Arrive in advance to discuss the clients and goals of the session with the clinician or supervisor. You also may be asked to attend a staffing before clients are seen. If you arrive late for a scheduled observation, you may not be allowed to observe. Entering late may disrupt the evaluation or management session. Tardiness is not responsible behavior.

3. **Introduce yourself to the clinical supervisor.** The clinical supervisor is responsible for his or her clients and their rights to privacy. The supervisor also is responsible for ensuring that you benefit from the clinical observation. Although observation was scheduled previously, there now may be reasons that prohibit the observation.

The client may have decided against being observed; the clinical supervisor may have determined that the observation area was too crowded or that the observation would not be beneficial for you or the client.

4. **Observe the entire clinical session.** When students observe only portions of clinical session, it is disruptive and decreases the value of the observation. Although clinical service varies according to the individual needs of clients and the personalities of the clinicians, all sessions have a certain progression. If you observe only portions of clinical sessions, you will not see the continuum of service delivery. For example, if you repeatedly arrive late, you may miss the client interview and, therefore, not understand why the clinician has chosen to administer specific tests. If you leave early, you may not know the results of the session and you will miss the closing interview.

5. **Do not interrupt the session or waste the clinician's preparation time.** Ask appropriate questions before and after sessions. Do not engage the clinician in irrelevant conversation. Clinicians are busy and usually have only a few minutes to prepare between clients.

6. **Maintain the client's privacy.** Client information is confidential. Do not discuss your observations with individuals outside the clinic setting. If it is necessary to discuss the client by name (e.g., with the clinician or clinical supervisor), do so only when you will not be overheard by others. To assure client confidentiality, avoid discussions in public areas. As part of the clinical learning experience, you will share information about your observations with other students. When you do so, do not refer to the client by name. Never remove information from a client's file or remove the client's folder from the clinical area.

7. **Act professionally.** Although you are a student and a guest in the clinical session, you represent the profession of audiology. You must present yourself as a professional in both attire and demeanor. Dress like a professional; do not wear shorts or other types of casual dress. Act professionally and communicate appropriately with the clinician and the clinical supervisor. Before speaking, carefully evaluate what you plan to say in front of clients and their families.

8. **Complete an observation report form for each client.** Each university has different record keeping and reporting procedures. Follow the procedures outlined by your department. Typically, you need to note the number of hours observed, what was observed, who was observed, and the location and date of the observation. The clinical supervisor then signs the form to verify the observation hours. You also may be required to complete an observation report detailing specific

aspects of each observation. Again, your university will supply you with any forms that are required.

Clinical Practicum

After you have completed the preclinic academic courses and 25 hours of supervised clinical observation, you may begin working with clients. You will gain experience with clients of different ages and with different communicative disorders. The majority of your clinical practicum will be completed in the area of audiology. You also will obtain some experience in screening, evaluating, and managing individuals with speech or language disorders as part of your speech-language pathology practicum requirement.

Supervision Requirements of Clinical Practicum

The ASHA Council on Professional Standards in Speech-Language Pathology and Audiology (1990) has outlined several requirements for supervision of clinical practicum. As with other ASHA guidelines, these requirements ensure a quality educational program. The following is an overview of supervision requirements.

1. **The clinical practicum supervisor must hold a current CCC.** There must be a clinical practicum supervisor with current CCC on site at both on- and off-campus sites at all times.

2. **The clinical practicum supervisor may provide supervision only in his or her area of certification.** In other words, an audiologist may not supervise speech-language pathology services, and a speech-language pathologist may not supervise audiological services. Exceptions to this are in the area of initial identification of communicative disorders. For example, both audiologists and speech-language pathologists may supervise screenings for communicative disorders. The audiologist may supervise screening of speech and language disorders, and the speech-language pathologist may supervise nondiagnostic audiologic screening.

3. **Supervision must be provided for 25% of each management session and 50% of each evaluation session.** Much of audiology practicum is diagnostic; therefore, the majority of your practicum may be supervised at least 50% of the time. As you progress in practicum, you will be able to work more independently; however, your supervisor will still be required to meet these minimum guidelines for frequency of supervision.

4. **The clinical practicum supervisor may include direct and indirect observation.** The majority of supervision will be direct observation. However, your supervisor also may observe your sessions by closed-circuit television. Regardless of the types of observation, or the amount of direct observation, your supervisor must evaluate your performance and give you feedback and direction to help you improve your clinical skills.

Additional information regarding the role of the clinical supervisor is covered in Chapter 4. Remember, these are minimum ASHA guidelines. In addition to the ASHA requirements, many states have additional licensure and credential requirements that clinical supervisors must meet.

Number of Clinical Clock Hours Required

ASHA describes clinical practicum requirements in terms of the number of clinical clock hours needed. Students working toward a CCC in Speech-Language Pathology or Audiology must complete a total of 375 clinical clock hours. Students applying for the CCC must have completed the following requirements (ASHA Clinical Certification Board, 1992):

1. **A minimum of 25 supervised clinical observation hours.** The 25 clinical observation hours must be completed prior to working with clients and must be supervised by the university staff or affiliates of the university. As you know, all clinical supervisors must hold a current CCC in their areas of supervision.

2. A minimum of **350 clock hours** with at least **250 of the hours earned in audiology practicum** at the graduate level.

3. A minimum of **50 clock hours earned in each of three types of clinical settings.** Although each clinical setting must offer a unique clinical experience, it is not always necessary for the clinical settings to be at different institutions. For example, your university may offer experience in pediatric audiology clinic, geriatric audiology clinic, and a clinic specializing in electrophysiological testing. Private practices, hospitals, public schools, physicians' offices, and other clinics also may offer experiences in multiple clinical settings. You may also fulfill this requirement at three different locations. Your clinical practicum may include experience at the university clinic, a Veteran's Administration hospital, and community hospital. Another student may complete practicum in the university clinic, a private practice, a military hospital, and a pediatric hospital. Clinical experience in distinctly separate locations often provides a more varied experience in terms

of different written and oral reporting requirements, time restrictions for client preparation and provision of services, and supervision. This variety may better prepare you for your future role as a professional audiologist.

4. A minimum of **40 clock hours earned in evaluation of hearing in children.**

5. A minimum of **40 clock hours earned in evaluation of hearing in adults.**

6. A minimum of **80 hours must be earned in the selection and use of amplification and assistive devices, with a minimum of 10 hours each with children and adults.**

7. A minimum of **20 clock hours earned in the management of hearing disorders in children and adults.**

8. A minimum of **35 clock hours in speech-language pathology.** These hours must be unrelated to hearing impairment and include 15 hours in evaluation or screening and 15 hours in management. The remaining 5 hours may be in evaluation, screening, or management.

9. A maximum of **20 optional clock hours may be earned in related disorders.** Related disorders include such activities as hearing conservation programs or intraoperative monitoring. These hours are not mandatory.

10. **Some experience with both individual and group client contact.**

The standards for individuals submitting applications for the CCC in Speech-Language Pathology are similar to the standards for Audiology applicants. Briefly, these standards require students to complete a minimum of 375 clock hours that include the following (ASHA Clinical Certification Board, 1992):

1. A minimum of **25 supervised clinical observation hours.**

2. A minimum of **350 total clinical practicum clock hours with a total of 250 of the hours earned at the graduate level in speech-language pathology.**

3. A minimum of **50 clock hours earned in each of three types of clinical settings.**

4. minimum of **20 evaluation hours in each of the following categories: speech disorders in children, speech disorders in adults, language disorders in children, and language disorders in adults.**

5. A minimum of **20 management hours in each of the following: speech disorders in children, speech disorders in adults, language disorders in children, language disorders in adults.**

6. A minimum of **35 hours in audiology.** Of these 35 hours, 15 hours are required in the evaluation or screening of auditory disorders, and 15 hours are required in the habilitation or rehabilitation of indi-

viduals with auditory disorders. The remaining 5 hours may be earned in either evaluation of auditory disorders or in the area of habilitation or rehabilitation of individuals with auditory disorders.

7. **Experience with both individual and group client contact.**

8. A maximum of **20 optional clock hours may be earned in related disorders.** Activities may include improved oral pharyngeal functioning, prevention of speech or language disorders, or development and conservation of optimal communication.

Your department may have additional practicum hour requirements. The total clock hours required by ASHA are the minimum number of practicum hours. To gain the maximum benefit from your training program, pursue as many practicum experiences as you can. Devote time to each experience. You may be surprised by how different clinical practicum experiences assist you in developing your clinical skills and knowledge and by how that skill and knowledge can be generalized across patients and settings. For example, if you are confident that you do not want to work with children, you may be hesitant to become fully involved in the pediatric clinic. However, in this clinic you may learn a variety of behavior management and observation skills that will help you wherever you work. Check with your advisor regularly to find out what clinical practicum positions are available and to ensure that you meet the requirements of ASHA and your university.

What to Count as Clinical Clock Hours

You will spend time preparing for clinical practicum and completing various requirements related to client service. However, much of this time cannot be counted as clinical clock hours. With few exceptions, only direct client contact is counted as clinical clock hours. Use the following guidelines in recording your clock hours (ASHA Clinical Certification Board, 1992):

1. **Count supervised clock hours earned in conjunction with a class assignment.** For example, as part of a class assignment you may be required to evaluate the hearing of five of your classmates. However, to count this time as clinical clock hours, 50% of the evaluation must have been supervised. Practice administering certain tests should not be counted.

2. **Count direct client contact clock hours earned in clinical practicum.**

3. **Count clock hours earned for counseling clients or counseling or training family members.**

4. **Count clock hours spent in obtaining or giving assessment and management information.** You can count the time you spend taking a case history, interviewing the client, the client's family, or both. You can also count the time you spend discussing your diagnosis and recommendations with the client or the client's family.

5. **Count the different services you provide separately.** The services you provide for one client may include many of the categories ASHA includes as part of its minimum clock hour requirements. For example, one client may require a hearing evaluation; hearing aid evaluation, fitting, training, and follow-up management sessions. Divide your clock hours according to how much time was spent in each area.

6. **Count a maximum of 25 clinical staffing hours as clock hours.** Clinical staffings include activities such as meetings with other professionals to discuss your client's management. However, meetings with your clinical supervisor to discuss management plans and procedures cannot be counted as clinical staffings. You may count the staffing hours as part of the required 375 clock hours; however, the staffing hours cannot be used to meet any of the minimum ASHA requirements. For example, you spent four hours related to evaluating an adult client's hearing. Of those four hours, three involved direct audiological evaluation and one involved staffing. Only the three hours of evaluation may be used to meet the minimum of 40 hours required in evaluation of hearing in adults.

7. **Do not count preparation time as clinical clock hours.** Although you will spend much time calibrating and preparing equipment, writing reports, developing management plans, and scoring tests, you cannot count clock hours for these activities. The majority of clinical practicum clock hours is earned for direct client contact time only. If you have questions regarding what to count as clock hours, ask your clinic supervisor.

Payment for Clinical Services

ASHA guidelines prohibit you from receiving payment for clinical services. However, you may be eligible for scholarships, grants, stipends, or other types of financial aid. Some practicum sites provide grants or stipends. These are not considered payment for clinical services, but are an incentive to attract exceptional students and an asset in defraying living expenses. Your university also may have scholarships, grants, or stipends for which you can apply. ASHA regularly publicizes scholarships available to students of communicative disorders. Your advisor and the financial aid office at your university can give you information on financial assistance available to you.

Clinical Practicum as a Learning Experience

Clinical practicum is a vehicle designed to supplement and enhance knowledge and skills acquired in academic course work. Although you will learn much information in your academic course work, clinical practicum gives you the opportunity to apply the information and experience the strengths, weaknesses, pros, and cons of the different theories and techniques you have studied.

Clinical practicum provides a unique learning experience. When you begin your clinical practicum, you are not expected to perform as a professional. You are expected to have an academic foundation on which you and your clinical supervisors can expand. Opportunities for learning arise as you see a wide variety of clients in different clinical settings.

You may be somewhat apprehensive about beginning your clinical practicum. This is not unusual. Many students are nervous when they first begin their clinical practicum assignments. Most quickly find that clinical practicum is a challenging but rewarding method of learning.

2
Organization of Clinical Practicum

To enhance students' learning and help them gain confidence, clinical practicum experiences are organized on a continuum of experience and skill levels. This continuum provides students with clinical experience based on their educational background and prior clinical involvement. Together with other aspects of clinical practicum, this continuum ensures quality patient care. Students begin their practicum assignments requiring maximum supervision when providing services for clients with less complex disorders and progress to requiring minimal supervision when providing services for clients with more complex diagnostic and intervention needs.

After you have completed 25 supervised clinical observation hours and other academic requirements, you will be eligible to begin your clinical practicum. Clinical practicum typically begins at the university clinic. During your first semester of clinical practicum, you may complete your speech-language pathology practicum requirements and begin your audiology practicum requirements.

As you know, audiology majors must complete 35 clinical clock hours of speech-language pathology practicum including a minimum of 15 evaluation hours and 15 management hours. You will be assigned one or two clients with relatively simple communication disorders. For instance, you may be assigned a child who demonstrates only a few isolated errors of articulation. You will evaluate and provide service for the client. You may be required to perform additional speech-language assessments or screenings to complete your evaluation hours.

Audiology students with heavy academic and clinical demands sometimes question the necessity of speech-language practicum. However, this practicum is mandated by ASHA. This brief introduction to speech-language pathology practicum may help you better understand and recognize normal and abnormal speech and language, as well as better understand the responsibilities of the speech-language pathologist. Also, both the client management and observation skills you acquire in your speech-language pathology practicum are useful in working with audiology clients.

As a beginning student clinician in audiology, you will have a less demanding clinical schedule than more advanced audiology student clinicians. You may be scheduled to see clients only 2 to 4 hours per week and, as much as possible, be assigned the clients with less complex needs. For example, initially, you may perform only standard pure-tone, immittance, and speech evaluations. As you gain experience, become more confident, and are able to make more independent decisions, your clinical schedule is increased and you will be assigned clients who require more complex assessment and management, including hearing aids. After you have completed 1 to 2 semesters of audiology practicum at the university clinic, your supervisor will determine if you are prepared to begin your off-campus clinical internships. Off-campus clinical internships vary in the prerequisite skills required and the clinical opportunities offered.

THE TYPICAL UNIVERSITY CLINIC

The typical university clinic serves a wide variety of individuals from the community. Both speech-language pathology and audiology services often are available. The university clinic is designed to provide quality clinical services for these individuals while maintaining necessary educational experiences for student clinicians. These educational experiences may include research activities as well as direct client services.

Supervision

Regular observation and supervision will be routine components of your university clinic experience. Student clinicians providing audiological services at a university clinic may be observed by supervisors, family members of clients, and other students. Remember, the majority of your clinical activities will be evaluative, and you will be supervised for at least 50% of each session. Your supervisor may determine that you require additional supervision based on factors such as the complexity of your client's disorder, the amount of your clinical experience, your academic background, your clinical skill level, or a combination of these factors. Your supervisor may observe you directly via an observation window or indirectly on closed-circuit television. It is not unusual for a supervisor to enter the room to demonstrate an assessment procedure or to observe your session more closely.

Occasionally, your sessions may be videotaped. Your supervisor may direct you to watch these tapes and observe certain procedures or specific clinical interactions. Some videotapes also may be used for class demonstrations. Videotaping is sometimes unsettling for beginning student clinicians. However, videotapes are excellent learning resources. Reviewing your session on videotape allows you to evaluate the session objectively. Videotaped sessions also allow students to observe clients and situations that they might not otherwise encounter.

You probably will have only one supervisor during your first term of clinical practicum. However, clinical scheduling and departmental policy regulate supervisor assignments. For instance, if you enroll in both speech-language pathology and audiology practicum, you will have at least two different clinical supervisors, one for speech-language pathology and one for audiology clinic. Your clinical supervisor may be a member of the university teaching faculty, full-time supervisory faculty, part-time supervisory staff, or a combination of the three.

In the past, there has been some confusion regarding the supervision requirements for hearing screening activities. ASHA considers identification audiometry associated with hearing conservation programs to be a diagnostic activity. As a diagnostic activity, it requires a minimum of 50% supervision. Many program supervisors consider 50% supervision of screening activities sufficient for the beginning practicum student. Few would consider 100% supervision of screening activities as necessary. Identification audiometry should be conducted only in a registered practicum under the supervision of the properly certified and licensed professional to ensure that practicum credit is received. Hearing screenings and practice testing conducted as a part of a class requirement, before students have completed their prerequisite 25 hours of observation, do not count toward clinical hours, even when supervised by appropriately certified and licensed personnel.

Supervision must be provided by an individual currently holding an ASHA Certificate of Clinical Competence in the area in which he or she supervises (speech-language pathology or audiology). If not prohibited by state licensure laws, speech-language pathologists may supervise nondiagnostic audiologic screenings as part of initial identification of a communicative disorder or as part of a speech and language evaluation. Audiologists also may supervise speech and language screenings as part of initial identification of a communicative disorder. Both audiologists and speech-language pathologists may supervise aural habilitative and rehabilitative services. Although acknowledging some supervision "overlap," ASHA directs that supervision in the minor areas be provided by an individual certified in that area (ASHA Clinical Certification Board, 1992). For example, although you (an audiology major) may earn some speech-language evaluation hours while screening your audiology patients' speech and language, the majority of your speech-language evaluation hours should be earned under the supervision of a certified speech-language pathologist.

Your supervisor routinely critiques your clinical skills in the form of verbal or written feedback. Your supervisor will identify both the strengths and weaknesses observed in your clinical performance and help you identify necessary changes. Eventually, your supervisor will expect you to learn to analyze and critique your own clinical sessions.

Clinic Schedules

University clinic schedules may be based on the academic schedule of the university. Therefore, the clinical services may be provided only 9 to 10 months of the year. This schedule can interrupt continuity of service and, without adequate planning, may result in hardship for clients with hearing aids that need repair. Other university clinics provide services throughout the year and are more easily able to meet client needs.

Speech-language pathology clients usually are scheduled for two to three sessions per week. Each session usually ranges from 30 to 60 minutes. Although most clients are seen individually, some clients may receive management in a group setting. As a beginning clinician, you will probably not be assigned to provide group services.

In contrast to speech-language pathology clients who often receive management for the entire semester, audiology clients may only be seen a few times each year. Many audiology clients require only a hearing evaluation and are seen once.

Audiology appointments vary according to the needs of the client and experience of the student clinician. Appointments for standard hearing evaluations may be scheduled for 1 to 2 hours. Time scheduled for hearing aid fittings, consultations, and other habilitative services varies depending on the complexity of the client's disorder as well as the dynamics of the client's family. During the appointment, you should obtain the client's history, perform the necessary assessments, review the results with the client, make recommendations, complete billing information, and assist the client in scheduling his or her next appointment. If a hearing aid has been recommended, you also may need to fill out the hearing aid order forms.

Because of the many components of audiology sessions, beginning student clinicians often need, and are allowed, more time to complete a session than more advanced student clinicians. Therefore, initially, you may evaluate 1 to 2 clients per day, 1 to 2 days per week. As you gain more experience, the number and variety of clients assigned to you gradually will be increased.

In addition to direct client contact, you may be required to attend staffings. As in audiology appointments, staffings vary in time depending on the number of clients being staffed, the complexity of the clients' disorders, and the experience of the student clinicians. You should probably plan to spend at least 1 hour per week for staffings.

At the beginning of the semester, you will be given your clinic schedule and assigned your clinical supervisor. In your speech-language pathology practicum, you may be responsible for telephoning the client and confirming the client's clinic schedule. In audiology clinic, your clients typically will be scheduled by the clinic secretary. It will be your responsibility to check the schedule in advance to make sure you are prepared and aware of any changes (such as cancellations) that have occurred.

Types of Clients

The types of clients seeking services at the university clinic are influenced by a variety of factors. The demographics of the area, clinic schedules, expertise of the faculty, adequate audiological equipment, and other audiology or speech-language pathology services available in the area all assist in determining the population served at the university clinic. Generally, the university clinic's caseload reflects a diverse range of ages and communicative disorders. However, there may be some exceptions to this. For example, if there is a large pediatric facility in the area, the audiology clinic may evaluate few infants and children.

The university speech and hearing clinic also is influenced by the department's relationship with allied health services at the university. For example, if there is a large otolaryngology training program at the university, the clinic may serve many of its clients.

Report Writing and Record Keeping

Audiology clinic requires students to be able to write quickly and succinctly. Reports may be required for each clinic appointment and often are due the day after the appointment. You may be required to use a computer or specific word processing program. Each clinic has different policies and terminology regarding writing assignments. You should review any questions you have regarding reporting format, due dates, and so on with your supervisor.

In addition to written reports, you will be required to report information in your client's chart. Generally, this information is very brief and refers the reader to the written report for more complete information.

Off-Campus Practicum Sites

After you have completed one to two semesters of clinical practicum at the university audiology clinic, you will be ready to begin off-campus practicum. Practicum sites vary depending on your university, the region you live in, and your career goals. Although you should have a variety of experiences, you also may want to focus your training in a specific area of interest.

Off-campus practicum sites include private and community hospitals, pediatric hospitals, Veteran's Administration hospitals, schools, private practices, and physicians' offices. Student clinicians planning to earn a credential to work in public schools also may be required to complete an internship in the public school setting.

An audiologist employed by the off-campus site provides the primary supervision of off-campus practicum. The supervisor must be ASHA-certified and meet appropriate state licensure requirements. Often, a university supervisor or clinic director consults with the site supervisor regarding the practicum experience and the student clinician's performance. All supervision must comply with ASHA guidelines on frequency of supervision, type of supervision and supervisory qualifications.

Usually, you will be required to follow the holiday schedule of your off-campus site instead of the schedule of the university. There will be certain other professional responsibilities and rules of conduct to which you will be expected to adhere. These responsibilities and rules may be different from those of the university, but should not conflict with principles of the university clinic or ASHA guidelines on service delivery. For example, your off-campus practicum site may have different procedures than the university clinic regarding the protection of client confidentiality. However, respect for client confidentiality is still enforced.

Your off-campus supervisor will discuss your performance with the university supervisor and may suggest a practicum grade. Ultimately, the university supervisor is responsible for your grade based on the department's performance criteria. If you have questions or concerns regarding any evaluation you receive, discuss them with your clinical supervisor.

Hospitals

Audiologists working in a hospital setting provide services to a variety of individuals. In many hospitals, the majority of patients is seen in outpatient clinics. However, hospitals are expanding their audiological services to patients admitted to their facilities. The hospital setting also provides students with the opportunity to work closely with allied health professionals. Some of the professionals you will often communicate with are otologists, otolaryngologists, primary care physicians, speech-language pathologists, and nurses. The activities of your practicum will depend on the organization of the hospital and the requirements of your individual practicum assignment.

Supervision

In most hospitals, supervision is provided by a staff audiologist. Depending on the structure of the audiology program, you may have more than one supervisor. The supervising audiologists must hold a current ASHA certification in audiology and usually must meet appropriate state licensure requirements. If you are the only audiology intern at the hospital, you may receive one-to-one supervision. If there are other audiology interns, supervision will be divided among the interns. Initially, 100% of your sessions probably will be supervised. As you gain experience, supervision may decrease to the minimum required by ASHA. In the university clinic, supervisors often post schedules of times they are available to discuss clinic with you. In the hospital setting, it probably will be your responsibility to seek out your supervisor. Occasionally, you may need to come in early or stay late to discuss clinical issues with your supervisor.

Clinic Schedules

In the hospital outpatient clinic, it is not uncommon for audiology appointments to be scheduled on the half hour. You may have only 30 minutes to establish rapport with your client, obtain a case history, evaluate your client's hearing, review the results and recommendations of the evaluation session with your client, note results in your client's file, and prepare for your next client. Student clinicians often find the rapid pace of off-campus practicum one of their biggest challenges. However, you quickly will learn that you are able to complete all or most of the necessary activities in the allotted time. You also will find that you may have appointment cancellations which give you time to catch up on your paper work during the day.

Inpatient schedules may vary based on the types of services with which you are involved. For example, if you are involved in intraoperative monitoring, your schedule will be based on the schedule of the surgeon and the length of the surgery. If you are screening the hearing of a patient in acute care, you may spend only a few minutes with the patient.

Hospitals often require audiologists to spend a certain number of hours in direct patient care. For example, the audiologist working 8 hours per day, may be assigned 5½ hours of direct client care with the remaining time allowed for preparation, paperwork, and consultation with other professionals. As a student intern you may not be expected to adhere strictly to this schedule. At first you may be given two to three clients per day. Your clinic schedule will be increased as you gain experience. By the end of your internship, you will be following the schedule of the staff audiologist.

Types of Clients

The types of clients you see will be based on the demographics of the hospital. Your clients may range in age from birth through adult, or if there is a large pediatric facility in the area, the vast majority of your clients may be adults. As previously noted, your clients may be in- or outpatients. Among the inpatients, you may see individuals who are ill or recovering from serious injury. For example, you may be responsible for monitoring a patient's hearing while he or she is receiving ototoxic drug therapy. In this case, you may perform pure-tone screening at the patient's bedside. If you are working at a hospital where cochlear implants or stapedectomies are performed, you will work with clients before and after surgery, administering pre- and post-surgical audiological tests. With cochlear implant patients you may be involved in extensive speech reception training.

After surgery, you will work closely with inpatients and their families in providing any appropriate communicative management. Later you may see the same clients in the outpatient setting where you will see many clients who need hearing evaluations and hearing aids. Tests frequently administered in the hospital setting include pure-tone tests, speech tests, immittance audiometry, auditory brainstem response (ABR) audiometry, otoacoustic emission (OAE) audiometry, and electronystagmography (ENG). You may be required to learn a different and abbreviated testing format than the one you used at the university clinic. However, these changes should not cause you too much trouble. Remember, although you generally have more time to evaluate a client at the university clinic, by the time you begin your hospital practicum you will have gained considerable experience and have a broad academic and clinical foundation on which to expand.

Allied Health Specialists

In the medical setting, you will learn to work as a member of a multidisciplinary team. You will work with other professionals such as otologists, otolaryngologists, orthodontists, social workers, nurses, and speech-language pathologists. You will share your assessment results and recommendations with other team members. This communication may occur during "rounds" or "staffings." You will learn the role of each team member in the care and habilitation of the patient. In hospital rounds, you and other team members will meet with the physician in charge. You may go with the physician to the patients' rooms or meet in a conference room to discuss the patients' present hearing levels and management plan. The physician leads the discussion and may give information about the patient or ask questions of individual team members. The roles of other specialists are discussed in greater detail in Chapter 5.

Report Writing and Record Keeping

As part of your clinical practicum experience, you will be required to document assessment results, recommendations, intervention, and patient progress. Different hospitals have different reporting formats. One may require that reports be dictated; others may require that reports be generated on a word processor. Your supervisor will give you directions regarding the specific requirements at your hospital practicum site.

One widely used means of communication among professionals in hospitals is through information reported in the patients' charts. Many medical abbreviations and symbols are used in medical charts. You will need to learn these to read the patients' charts adequately and effectively write information in the charts. There are many references for medical abbreviations and symbols. Some of the commonly used medical abbreviations and symbols are listed in Appendix A.

Generally, you have little time to write reports and make notations in patients' charts. Also, other professionals do not have much time to read your reports. You will learn to write fast and concisely.

Pediatric Hospitals

The pediatric hospital is designed to serve children. As much as possible, the facilities are decorated and furnished to help make children and their families feel comfortable. The size of equipment may be appropriate for children. Many of your responsibilities as a student audiologist in the pediatric hospital will be similar to those performed in the community hospital setting. The following sections outline some of these similarities as well as some of the differences.

Supervision

Again, your supervisor will be an audiologist holding current ASHA certification in audiology. Unlike the community hospital setting, your supervisor may be closely involved in helping you develop skills in behavior control. Also, because many of your clients will be young toddlers, you will need to learn to perform tests that give you the most useful information first and perform them rapidly. Your supervisor may suggest shortcuts or model certain testing skills you need to develop.

Your supervisor also will help you develop your counseling skills. You will be working with families who may be facing the possibility of having a child who has a disability. Family members may display many emotions including grief, hostility, guilt, and denial. On the positive side, you will work with families who are relieved and happy to find out either that their children's hearing abilities are normal or that there are many ways to help their children with whatever type of hearing problem they have.

Clinic Schedules

Although your appointments may be scheduled for 60-minute intervals, you may finish in 30 to 40 minutes because of your clients' ability (or lack of ability) to attend to tasks. Also, your clients may fatigue quickly because of their ages or medical handicaps. You may obtain an abbreviated case history to decrease the amount of time the child has to wait before testing begins. As previously noted, you will perform tests quickly. You may begin with fast objective tests like otoacoustic emission and immittance testing and progress to speech reception tests and test a wide range of frequencies, rather than initially attempting to obtain behavioral thresholds for each frequency. At the end of the session, you will review your results and recommendations with your supervisor and then with your clients' parent or care provider.

Appointments often are scheduled to begin between 8:30 and 9:00 A.M. As in the community hospital setting, appointments are scheduled for approximately 5 to 6 hours of the work day. The remaining time can be used for consultation with other professionals and report writing.

Types of Clients

The large majority of your clients will be children, although pediatric hospitals also may provide services to certain adults to supplement their client base. For example, a client who was previously hospitalized for a head injury as a child may continue as a client at the hospital as an adult. The hospital also may provide services to adults with developmental delays. In some areas, pediatric audiology departments also serve the general community. For example, in addition to specializing in services for children, the pediatric audiology department may evaluate individuals seeking disability compensation for a hearing loss and screen employees for hearing conservation.

You may have clients who require pure-tone tests, speech tests, immittance, or electrophysiologic tests. Other clients may require central auditory processing tests. You may see in- and outpatients, with the majority of your patients being outpatients. Examples of clients seen in the inpatient setting include those served by cleft palate or cochlear implant teams. In the outpatient setting, you may see clients who have chronic ear infections, suspected hearing losses, or possible learning disabilities. You also may provide management services. In the pediatric hospital, you will work with many children, each of whom has a different personality and offers a different learning experience.

Allied Health Specialists

In all settings, it is important to provide comprehensive client services. In the pediatric setting, it is essential that comprehensive client services be provided. Many hospitals have special teams designed to meet the needs of their pediatric population. If the hospital has a large audiology department, one audiologist may serve on the cleft palate team, one on the genetics team, another on the cochlear implant team, and still another on the learning disabilities team. If the hospital has a small audiology department, one audiologist may serve on all of the multidisciplinary teams. Allied health professionals you may work with in the pediatric hospital include the otolaryngologist, pediatrician, dentist, orthodontist, psychologist, geneticist, nurse, social worker, speech-language pathologist, and special education teacher. See Chapter 5 for more information regarding the roles of these professionals.

Report Writing and Record Keeping

Basically, report writing and record keeping requirements in a pediatric hospital are the same as those in the community hospital. However, because many of your reports may be used in the public school setting, some of your recommendations may change. For example, you may need to use caution in recommending aural rehabilitation 5 days a week for a child who will receive services in a public school. To become familiar with the vocabulary and abbreviations used in the pediatric hospital, you might want to refresh your memory regarding common childhood illnesses and common childhood traumas. This may help you in understanding other individuals' reports.

Public Schools

Requirements for working as an audiologist in the public schools differ across states. In some states, audiologists must obtain a credential or certificate to provide services in the public schools. Student clinicians may be required to complete a practicum experience in a school setting or to obtain a minimum number of hours working with school-age children. If you are interested in working in the public schools, discuss your state's requirements with your advisor.

Supervision

As in all clinical practicum settings, the student clinician providing services in the public schools must be supervised by an audiologist with a current CCC in audiology. In addition to complying with appropriate state licensure requirements, the supervisor also may be required to hold a special credential or certificate to provide services and supervise student clinicians in the public schools. Evaluation sessions must be supervised at least 50% of the time and management sessions at least 25% of the time. Because audiologists working in school systems often travel to several different schools per day, it is important to remember that a person with current CCC-A must be on site before you may provide any service. For example, your supervisor might ask you to meet him at Jefferson School at 1:00 P.M. You arrive at 1:00 P.M. and discover that your supervisor is going to be 5 to 10 minutes late. According to ASHA guidelines, you are not allowed to begin service delivery until a qualified supervisor is on site.

Clinic Schedules

Schools usually begin around 8:00 A.M. and end any time from 11:30 A.M. for kindergartners or preschoolers to 4:00 P.M. for high school students.

Again, depending on the demographics of the school district and the types of services you are scheduled to provide, you may be assigned to one school or, more likely, to travel to many different schools.

Types of Clients

Audiology services in the public schools are designed to meet the needs of all individuals who have a hearing handicap and are eligible for school services as mandated by federal legislation, The Education of All Handicapped Children's Act (EHA), Public Law (P.L.) 94-142 was passed on November 25, 1975. P.L. 94-142 is one of the cornerstones of contemporary special education. P.L. 94-142 mandated educational services for all handicapped children (Dublinske & Healey, 1978). Since 1975, several amendments to the EHA have been made and reauthorization of the discretionary programs of the EHA in 1990 changed the name of the EHA to Individuals with Disabilities Education Act (IDEA) (*ASHA Governmental Affairs Review,* 1990). Audiologists employed by the public school are governed by both federal laws and guidelines. In addition to following commonly accepted standards of practice, the school audiologist must also know and adhere to guidelines affecting their school sites.

A wide range of services is offered for children with disabilities in the public schools. School audiologists serve children of different age groups and children with hearing impairments ranging from mild to profound.

ASHA's position statement on audiology services in the schools (ASHA, 1993a) defined the service needs of children with hearing impairments in the schools as prevention, identification, assessment, rehabilitation and instructional services, follow-up, referral and monitoring, technical assistance and support, and evaluation and research. Within this scope of practice, ASHA (1993a) has listed the following 13 activities the school audiologist is qualified to perform and might be involved in.

1. Develop a high risk registry in conjunction with local medical personnel.
2. Organize and supervise a hearing screening program.
3. Train audiometric technicians to screen hearing.
4. Perform follow-up and threshold hearing tests.
5. Make appropriate referrals for further assessment.
6. Interpret assessment results to other school personnel.
7. Act as a member of the educational team and make recommendations about placement, communication needs, and modifica-

tion of classroom environments for the deaf and hard of hearing.
8. Educate parents, children, and school personnel about ways to prevent hearing impairment.
9. Make recommendations about use of personal and group amplification.
10. Monitor hearing aids and auditory training units and train others to do so.
11. Analyze classroom noise and make recommendations as to how to reduce its effects.
12. Calibrate audiometric equipment.
13. Serve as a liaison between the school and parents, teachers and special support personnel, and the school and relevant community agencies.

You might be surprised to learn that the audiologist working in the schools often is not the primary person responsible for performing audiometric screenings. According to a survey by Wall, Naples, Buhrer, and Capodanno (1985), audiometric screening was performed by technicians in 22.14% of the schools sampled; by nurses in 65.15% of the schools; speech-language pathologists in 33.58% of the schools; by parents, aides, or volunteers in 19.10% of the schools; and by audiologists in only 15.79% of the schools. One reason for this is because there are no universal standards for audiometric screeners. Another reason is that some school districts employ only one audiologist to provide services for a school district of 50,000 children. Obviously, in this case the audiologist needs to be involved in the more complex cases and will need assistance from an individual trained in administering and implementing a screening program.

Allied Health and Educational Specialists

As a student audiologist in the public school setting, you may be involved in individual education program (IEP) meetings involving the parents and other specialists in the schools. You will learn to work cooperatively with many other professionals including teachers, nurses, physicians, speech-language pathologists, psychologists, and principals. You also will learn new terminology in your school assignment. Appendix B contains a list of acronyms and abbreviations frequently used in the educational setting.

Report Writing and Record Keeping

In addition to writing the familiar clinical reports, you also may be involved in contributing to a child's IEP. In your school internship, you will learn to write management objectives using educational terms, relating these objectives to classroom performance. Your supervisor will give you writing guidelines.

Private Clinics

Many audiologists are in private practice. Private practices may be an integral part of an otolaryngologist's office, part of a joint speech-language pathology and audiology service, or a free-standing audiology office. In addition to being competent audiologists, professionals in private practice also must be versed in good business practices. They need to know how to start and run a business. They should have skills in accounting procedures, marketing their services, and maintaining good public relations. Private practitioners provide audiology services in their offices, and they often contract to provide audiological services with other agencies such as skilled nursing facilities, home health care agencies, and hospitals without audiology departments.

As a student clinician working in a private practice, you will develop skills in assessing and managing hearing disorders, as well as gain insight into the business aspects of your profession. You will learn about getting reimbursed by insurance companies and governmental programs such as Medicaid.

Supervision

Because the private practitioner is dependent on favorable public relations, your supervisor will closely supervise and give feedback on not only your technical skills, but also your interpersonal skills. Your supervisor will comply with all of ASHA's guidelines on clinical supervision of student clinicians.

Clinic Schedules

The private practice schedule often revolves around the schedules of the clients. For example, appointments may be scheduled on an hourly basis from 8:00 A.M. to 5:00 P.M.; however, clients having trouble with their hearing aids who drop by without an appointment are usually fitted into the schedule. Some practices schedule 45 minutes for evaluation and counseling of a client and leave 15 minutes of each hour available for additional or last-minute clients. Also, to serve clients who are unable to leave work, some private practices also make appointments before 8:00 A.M., after 5:00 P.M., or on Saturdays. Your schedule will depend on the schedule of your practicum site.

Types of Clients

Clients in a private practice may range in age from infants to elderly individuals. The entire range of communicative disorders may be managed in most private settings. However, you may be assigned to a private practice that specializes in pediatrics or geriatrics. You will perform hearing evaluations that include pure-tone tests, immittance tests, speech tests, electrophysiologic tests, and central auditory processing tests. You will counsel clients regarding their hearing, make appropriate recommendations, and prescribe and troubleshoot hearing aids. Students planning a practicum assignment in a private practice need to have a comprehensive knowledge of hearing aids. You also may be involved in hearing conservation.

Allied Health Specialists

In the private practice setting, you will communicate with a variety of professionals, although you primarily will work independently under the guidance of your supervisor. You will communicate with physicians, speech-language pathologists, and other audiologists. To a large extent, the type and frequency of communication with other specialists will depend on the private practice. For example, if you are working in a practice that is affiliated with an ear, nose, and throat specialist, you will have regular communication with that specialist. Many of your communications will be verbal, rather than written. If you are affiliated with speech-language pathologists, you may receive referrals from them and communicate with them on a regular basis regarding both the clinical and business needs of the practice. If you are at a practice run solely by audiologists, much of your communication with other professionals may be via short letters or reports, or some telephone calls.

Report Writing and Record Keeping

By necessity, both report writing and record keeping are quick and concise. You will have little time during the business day to write lengthy reports. Each office will have different forms of report writing and record keeping. Each office also will have different client billing procedures and paperwork handling in ordering hearing aids. Your supervisor will assist you in learning the necessary formats.

Veterans Administration Hospitals

Clinical practicum in the Veteran's Administration (VA) hospital will be similar to practicum in other hospital settings. One difference, of course, is that you will be working with veterans and, occasionally, with families of veterans. You will evaluate hearing, recommend hearing aids, counsel patients and patients' families, and provide all related audiological services for individuals with hearing impairment. You also may be called on to evaluate hearing in individuals seeking compensation on the basis of hearing loss. Some of these individuals may have nonorganic hearing losses. The nonorganic hearing loss may be further classified as **psychogenic** or **malingering.** Psychogenic hearing loss results from emotional trauma, usually accompanying temporary traumatic hearing loss. Malingerers are not found only in the military. However, student clinicians who have never encountered a malingerer before may meet one in the VA setting. A *malingerer* is an individual who claims to have more hearing loss than he or she actually has. In your audiology practicum you will learn the procedures use to identify and evaluate this type of individual.

Other Clinical Settings

Many other clinical settings are available to the student clinician. Opportunities for clinical experience are limited only by your imagination. Many universities encourage students to contact audiologists in the area to establish new internship sites. Some universities also allow students to complete internships in different cities. If you wish to gain practicum experience in a new setting, discuss your interest with your supervisor, clinical director, or academic advisor.

Clinical Internships

Practicum experiences in both on- and off-campus sites may be limited. Internships are a type of practicum that provides a comprehensive clinical experience for students. Qualified students generally are eligible to begin clinical internships after one to two semesters of on-campus clinical practicum. Clinical internships typically allow students a more "real-life" understanding of the demands of their future profession. Not only is direct patient management addressed in the clinical internship, but also indirect activities related to patient service and interpersonal relationships with other professionals can be developed more fully. Internships commonly are completed at off-campus sites such as hospitals, private practices, ENT offices, or schools.

Your internship assignment will be based on different factors. First, your clinical and academic experiences will determine whether you are qualified to begin an internship at a certain site. Some sites require students to have a minimum number of clinical hours and completed certain course work before beginning an internship at their site. Your supervisor also may make recommendations regarding your ability to perform required tasks at an internship site. Second, your clinical interests will influence the internships you are interested in applying for. For example, if you are interested in educational audiology, you may want to complete an internship in a public school. Third, your ability to travel and devote time to an internship will contribute to your consideration of different internships. Some students may elect to travel to a large hospital away from the university. Other students will select local internships. Students also may have the option of choosing part- or full-time internships.

Part-Time Internships

Student clinicians sometimes have scheduling options for their clinical practicum. Daily part-time internships are closely aligned with the requirements of a full-time internship, but allow students to schedule classes and work around the practicum assignment. While completing a part-time internship, students may work either a few hours a day or a few days each week. As previously noted, the type of internship you participate in will be determined by a variety of factors and will depend heavily on the needs and requirements of the practicum setting.

A part-time internship may benefit beginning student clinicians who need time to integrate information and have somewhat limited clinical skills. Experienced student clinicians who already have acquired knowledge and understanding of the many interpersonal abilities, managerial skills, and written and oral communication skills also may benefit from a part-time internship. A part-time internship is attractive to students because it allows some scheduling flexibility. However, students completing a part-time practicum assignment sometimes miss experiencing the full range interpersonal, professional, and business management aspects of a site. Students also may not fully experience the continuity of care in part-time clinical assignments. It is important to realize that some part-time practicum experiences may be so limited that you will not learn much about the setting and the clients served there. Carefully discuss your strengths, weaknesses, and needed clinical experience with your advisor.

Full-Time Internships

Full-time internships allow students to gain a comprehensive practicum experience. The full-time clinical internship may include both observation and clinical experiences. In addition to direct patient contact, you also may provide staff inservices and be included in rounds or staffings. During your full-time internship you will experience the daily routines and pressures associated with a particular setting and obtain a better understanding of the personal as well as professional requirements of the work setting. In a practicum, you often do not have this opportunity because you are not on site long enough. Students sometimes think that experiences and information not directly related to evaluation of hearing or hearing management are not necessary to their education. However, understanding the related requirements of your job will help make your first year as a professional easier and more successful. In addition, a good employee is more than a competent clinician, and the skills of a good employee often are developed in interactions outside the test booth. Student clinicians follow the same work schedule as the professionals employed at the practicum site. For example, if you are assigned to a hospital practicum site as a full-time intern, you probably will be required to arrive at work at 8:00 A.M. and work until 5:00 P.M., Monday through Friday, for a certain number of weeks or until you earn a specific number of clinical hours. If a school holiday does not coincide with the holidays of the practicum site, you will be expected to adhere to the schedule of the practicum site and not that of the university.

Discuss your internship interests with your advisor early in your graduate program. You will need to know the academic requirements of certain practicum sites and what times of the day your university offers classes that you might take concurrently with your internship.

General Administrative Procedures

There are many administrative procedures that must be followed to provide efficient and effective clinical services. For example, the training program must offer appropriate supervision by qualified professionals, ensure that facilities are safe and equipment is current and in working order, and maintain accurate clinical records. Clinics accredited by the Public Service Board (PSB) of ASHA have established some form of quality improvement process to document the various administrative procedures. Your university will give you specific information regarding the requirements in your department. The following is an overview of some administrative procedures.

Supervisor Qualifications

In addition to holding current certification from ASHA, supervisors must meet appropriate state licensure requirements. It is the department's responsibility to verify that supervisors have met certification and licensure requirements before students are placed under their supervision.

Besides meeting the certification requirements, supervisors must have other skills, such as the ability to discuss clinical issues and give clear instructions to student clinicians. One of the primary responsibilities of the clinical supervisor is to help students develop their clinical skills. This may include activities such as direct instruction, modeling, or assigned readings. Most universities have a supervisor evaluation procedure. At the end of each clinical assignment, students have the opportunity to evaluate their supervisors anonymously. These evaluations are confidential and designed to aid supervisors in determining their own strengths and weaknesses. Routine peer reviews also provide constructive feedback to the clinical supervisor. The roles of the supervisor and student clinician are discussed in detail in Chapter 4.

Facilities And Equipment

It is the training program's responsibility to ensure that both on- and off-site facilities are appropriate for students. The facility must be safe and clean. Training facilities must provide a professional environment with access to current, well-maintained equipment, appropriate tests, and necessary supplies. Calibration of equipment must be performed and documented according to current American National Standards Institute (ANSI) standards. Part of your clinic responsibility may be to perform daily listening checks of equipment, clean equipment, restock supplies, and generally maintain the clinic space.

The clinic also should have some form of clinical review to ensure quality service to its clients. This may include activities such as surveying client satisfaction, review of client folders for documentation of service, review of clinical recommendations, review of calibration logs, supervisor evaluations, and student-clinician evaluations.

In addition to ensuring that the on-campus clinic meets specific requirements, the training program is responsible for ensuring that off-campus sites meet minimum standards for student placement. Before you are placed at an off-campus practicum site, the training program evaluates many factors. These include the general facilities, supervisor qualifications and certification status, amount of supervision available, number and types of clients served, and approximate number of clinical hours students can earn at the site. The clinic director or audiology instructor may visit newly contracted facilities. Sometimes, a facility may appear to be appropriate for student placement, when, in fact, it is not. If you have any concerns about on- or off-campus facilities, do not hesitate to discuss them with your clinic director or advisor.

Clinic Fees

Clinic fees generate the money necessary to cover overhead costs, including rent, utilities, equipment, supplies, and salaries. Facilities that have been subsidized in the past are being required to generate income to cover their own costs and often to help cover the costs of non-income-generating services. For example, a hearing and speech clinic in a hospital may be required to cover its own costs and to contribute to the overhead generated by nursing, housekeeping, and other non-income-generating services. Many university clinics began as subsidized clinics. As resources in higher education shrink, more university speech and hearing clinics are required to charge fees to cover much of their overhead.

University Clinics

Many university speech and hearing clinics charge fees for clinical services provided. The fees usually do not cover the entire cost of client services but help cover some of the costs of clinic materials, supplies, and equipment. Generally, the fees charged by university clinics are nominal in comparison to fees charged at hospitals and private practices. However, the fee structure introduces student clinicians to billing procedures. Also, the fees make the service more valuable to clients. It sometimes seems that clients are more likely to keep and be on time for appointments that they pay for. At some clinics, fees are implemented on a fixed scale. Other clinics may offer services on a sliding fee scale. Still other clinics may waive fees for clients unable to afford payment. Before you work with clients, your supervisor will discuss the clinic's fee structure with you.

Each university will have procedures for informing clients and potential clients about the clinic fees. It is usually appropriate for you to inform your clients about the clinic's fee schedule. However, you have neither the responsibility, nor the authority, to reduce or waive fees. Refer clients or parents who ask questions about fees, waivers, payment plans, and so forth to the clinic office.

Other Clinics

Because Veteran's Administration hospitals are not fee-for-service institutions, they have downsized services in hearing and speech as money budgeted has not kept pace with services needed. Community hospitals and community speech and hearing centers of various types also have downsized some services to control overhead and increased fees to cover remaining overhead. Private audiology services must charge fees that will cover overhead and provide income for the audiologists or those services will go out of business. Charging fees is necessary to maintain services.

In off-campus practicum sites, fees are collected by front office personnel. Special arrangements for paying fees are worked out with the clinic director. Different facilities have different expectations for practicum students regarding fees. Some do not allow professional staff and students in practicum to discuss fees with clients. Other facilities require the student to be familiar with the fee structure, to inform the client regarding fees, to be familiar with insurance coverages, to be familiar with referral protocols for insurance coverage, and other issues related to fees for service. You will be told of the facilities expectations regarding fees early in your off-campus practicum experience.

Health Insurance

Many health insurance groups restrict services to a group of approved providers and will cover the full cost of services provided by physicians but only some or none of the cost of the same services provided by nonphysicians. Students should be aware of health care insurance requirements as they pertain to the facility in which the practicum is being conducted and to the individual patients being served. The following are important questions to ask:

1. Does the client have insurance that will cover all or part of the services rendered?
2. Does the client's insurance require approval for services prior to the delivery of services?
3. Does the client's insurance allow payment for services delivered by a student in training?
4. Does the facility process insurance claim forms for the patient?

These issues often are covered by the practicum supervisor in the early stages of the practicum experience. Take notes and refer to them until you are comfortable that you know the procedures of your practicum facility.

Scheduling Practicum Assignments

Your practicum will be assigned and scheduled based on factors such as your clinical and academic experience, the number of clinical clock hours you need, your specific areas of interest, the availability of practicum sites, the number of clients seeking services, and the availability of clinical supervisors. To be able to communicate your practicum needs clearly to your advisor, maintain an accurate record of the clinical hours you have earned and the clinical hours you need to meet your university's requirements. Also, discuss with your advisor any specific clinical experiences you may want to pursue. You may want to visit different sites before deciding to request a specific assignment. Because of the many variables involved in making clinical assignments, it is important for you to adhere to the department's procedures for clinic assignments and to communicate regularly with the clinic director or other individuals in charge of scheduling.

Student Records

The clinic staff maintains student clinicians' records. These records include a variety of documents such as clinic application forms, performance reports, and documentation of clinical hours earned. All of these forms become part of your permanent clinical record and must be kept current by you and the clinic staff. ASHA site visitors routinely review student clinicians' files during the accreditation process.

Before you are admitted into clinical practicum, you will be required to complete certain forms. Questions on these forms generally ask for some biographical, academic, employment, and volunteer information. You also will need to provide documentation concerning certain pre-clinic requirements such as completion of clinical observation hours, insurance coverage, and current vaccinations. All of this information is maintained in your student-clinician file.

Prior to beginning your clinical practicum, the clinic staff will review your records to ensure you have met all the prerequisites for clinical practicum. As you earn clinical practicum clock hours, verification of these hours will be placed in your clinical file. It is important to maintain complete and accurate records of your clinical experience. Clinical clock hours earned should be accurately reported under the correct category, and the reporting form should be signed by your clinical supervisor. Other information relevant to your clinical practicum, such as clinical evaluations and letters of recommendation, also will be placed in your clinic file. Your clinic records are reviewed periodically to ensure that they meet both university and ASHA guidelines for clinical practicum, including the types of patients served and number of clinical hours earned.

Periodically, review your file to make sure the information is accurate. You may want to keep copies of your evaluations and clinical clock hours in your own files for comparison.

Clinic Supplies, Materials, And Equipment

During your clinical practicum, you will use a variety of supplies, materials, and equipment. These items are essential to your clinical service delivery, and many of them will be provided by the university clinic or off-campus site. Many university clinics require student clinicians to pay lab fees to cover the use of consumable items, such as test response forms. In some cases, you also may be required to purchase manuals of various tests and other procedures.

Clinic inventory can be divided into three general categories: supplies, materials, and equipment. Supplies are consumable items such as tongue depressors, gauze, cotton swabs, gloves, finger cots, tissues, batteries, disinfectant, cotton or sponge ear dams, and other items used to make earmolds. Materials also are categorized as consumable or expendable items, but often may be re-used many times before being replaced. Tests, books, toys, immittance probe tips, otoscope speculums, and procedure manuals often are classified as clinic materials. Clinical equipment is not consumable and is nonexpendable. It is generally more expensive than supplies and materials and used over a long period of time. Clinical equipment includes audiometers, computers, tape recorders, sound level meters, auditory trainers, otoscopes, stethoscopes, and augmentative communication devices.

Although you may not be required purchase your own supplies, materials, or equipment, it is important for you to take care of them. Following are some general guidelines.

1. Do not needlessly waste supplies. Use the supplies necessary to provide quality client service. Replace unused supplies in the appropriate containers and notify the clinic secretary if new supplies need to be ordered.
2. Use equipment according to the manufacturers' guidelines. For example, warm up equipment if directed to do so by the manufacturer, or turn off equipment not in use.
3. Clean all equipment and materials immediately. Make sure that your clinic room is clean and orderly and that all equipment and materials are properly cleaned before leaving at the end of the day.
4. Avoid rough handling of equipment. If you accidentally drop equipment such as headphones, make sure they are still working correctly before using them or putting them away.
5. Promptly report broken equipment. If you discover that certain equipment is broken or not working correctly, notify the individual responsible for equipment operation and maintenance.

In addition to these general guidelines, there will be specific instructions you must follow for different types of equipment. These instructions typically are found in the equipment manuals. Your supervisor or clinic director may provide additional information on the use, care, and maintenance of special clinical or research equipment you use.

3

The Conduct of the Student Clinician

Many characteristics distinguish effective audiologists. They should have knowledge about hearing and its disorders and skills in assessing and managing those disorders. Also, professional audiologists should maintain a certain professional standard of behavior and abide by rules of ethics established by their professional associations. Through course work and clinical practicum, student clinicians acquire these characteristics of effective audiologists. Clinical practicum is especially designed to have the students learn certain standards and ethics of practice. Different aspects of professional behavior and the various codes and regulations governing this behavior will be discussed in this chapter.

General Professional Behavior

Certain behaviors are universally accepted as appropriate for professionals. You should learn to incorporate these behaviors into your performance and demeanor early in your clinical practicum. As a student clinician, you are a representative of the university department, the university clinic, and the university at large. You, and your supervisor, may be the only professionals some of your clients ever receive audiological services from. To these clients, you and your supervisor will be the sole representatives of the entire profession of audiology. As you progress through your clinical practicum, you will contact and interact with many clients and professionals. Some of your communications will be in writing, but many will be through personal contact or telephone communication. Obviously, the importance of developing professional skills and behaviors as well as technical skills cannot be overemphasized.

Specific areas of conduct are outlined in the Code of Ethics of the American Speech-Language-Hearing Association (ASHA). In addition to these specific mandates, there are general rules of professional behavior. Some of these general rules, such as punctuality in meeting clinic deadlines, working cooperatively with others, being well prepared for assignments, and assuming responsibility for clinic equipment and facilities, probably are not dissimilar to rules you had to follow throughout your academic career, from kindergarten through college. You will also be expected to maintain appropriate dress and demeanor. Professional demeanor is a somewhat elusive term, but suggests that you are confident of your abilities and able to communicate in an organized, mature, and effective manner; establish rapport with clients; utilize clinical appointment time effectively; dress appropriately; and exhibit respect for your client, yourself, and your supervisor. This is one of the initial variables on which you are judged.

As a student clinician, you will work with many different clients. You probably will be nervous, especially during your first semester of clinical practicum, but through a combination of your demeanor and clinic performance, you must make the client believe that you are capable of providing quality clinical services. Several things contribute to earning the trust of the client. You may have exceptional clinical skills; but, if you are not able to establish rapport with your client, the client may not feel you are competent and be uncomfortable with your diagnosis and recommendations. Some of the means of establishing the trust and relationship between the client and clinician may be quite superficial, such as the way you dress or the way you wear your hair. Other factors are more objective, such as the amount of eye contact you make or the firmness of your handshake. Still other variables may be more elusive to pinpoint, such as your congeniality or ability to express empathy with your client. Again, as a student clinician, you are not expected to know everything. Your supervisor is there to help you. You should ask questions when you need help, and certainly, you should never pretend to know how to perform an unfamiliar procedure. However, it is important for you to present yourself as a person confident in his or her skills. The better prepared you are for each clinical experience, the easier it will be for you to appear confident, even when you may be slightly nervous.

Administrators, employees, and clients at off-campus sites may have little direct interaction with the university or your university department. Basically, you represent the university. Both your clinical performance and your professional behavior will influence the off-campus site's evaluation of your university training program. Before you begin practicum at an off-campus site, your university supervisor, advisor, or clinic director will determine if you have the necessary prerequisite skills to begin practicum off-campus. Certain off-campus sites may also interview you or review your clinical training before accepting you as a student clinician. However, once you have accepted an off-campus assignment, it is your responsibility to continue to be as well-prepared for each assignment as possible. You are expected to be punctual, maintain regular attendance, and learn new information by independent research as well as through assistance from your clinic supervisor. Although you are not expected, initially, to know all the procedures and regulations of a practicum site, you are expected to behave professionally. You should know that each site has certain professional policies and procedures, that policies and procedures may vary from site to site, and that it is your responsibility to find out and adhere to these policies and procedures. For instance, a practicum site may have particular procedures for reporting an absence due to illness or a formal method for communicating with allied professionals.

In both your on- and off-campus practicum experiences, you are expected to learn and adhere to many policies and procedures. Before you begin your on-campus clinical practicum, you will also study the ASHA Code of Ethics.

ASHA Code of Ethics

Both professionals and student clinicians must adhere to the Code of Ethics. As a student clinician, and in the future as a practicing audiologist, you will face situations where you must determine the most appropriate and ethical clinical action. While you are a student clinician, your clinical supervisor and your clinic policy manual will guide you in making clinical decisions. Both your supervisor's actions and the clinic's policies and procedures are based on the ASHA Code of Ethics and various ASHA position statements. As a professional, you will rely on the Code of Ethics, position statements, guidelines, and communications with colleagues. Official position statements, guidelines, and reports are published (ASHA, 1990a-b, 1991a-b, 1992b-c, 1993b-c). However, as a professional in private practice or as an employee, you will have the additional responsibility of making ethical judgments with the pressure of showing a financial profit. This is unavoidable. Of course, you want to make money, and your employer wants to profit from having you as an employee. As a student clinician, you may not be influenced by financial profit or loss, but you will be influenced by how your clinical and educational performance appears to your supervisor. To preclude your professional behavior or judgment being adversely influenced by financial or educational pressure, it is important for you to know ASHA's Code of Ethics and position statements. You also may want to evaluate your own value system and related behaviors to determine if they are consistent with the intent of the Code of Ethics.

Many professional organizations have a Code of Ethics defining appropriate behavior for their members. ASHA is no different. The ASHA Code of Ethics was developed by ASHA and approved by its legislative council. The Code of Ethics has been revised several times to meet the changing standards of practice. ASHA's Council on Professional Ethics in Speech-Language Pathology and Audiology is responsible for suggesting changes needed in the Code of Ethics. The Code of Ethics was designed to provide a standard of professional behavior that members of the audiology and speech-language pathology professions are expected to uphold. The Code of Ethics is not a legal document. Except in states that have adopted the Code of Ethics as part of licensure requirements, the code has no legal basis. Nonetheless, the code has been adopted by ASHA and its members as a standard of professional behavior. A professional who violates the Code of Ethics faces disciplinary action by ASHA's Ethical Practice Board (EPB). The EPB is responsible for the administration and enforcement of the code. When you apply for ASHA certification, you agree to uphold and abide by ASHA's Code of Ethics. Members of ASHA who fail to comply with the Code of Ethics face disciplinary action by the EPB. Examples of disciplinary action may include loss or suspension of an individual's ASHA certification, membership in ASHA, or both.

Both as a student clinician and, in the future, as an audiologist, you will want to comply with ASHA's Code of Ethics as part of your professional responsibility. You will find that many employers require that their audiologists hold current ASHA certification, and, as you now know, failing to comply with the code could result in suspension or loss of your ASHA certification.

The ASHA Code of Ethics includes a Preamble, and four Principles of Ethics. Each Principle of Ethics is subdivided into numerous Rules of Ethics. The Principles of Ethics are general statements suggesting the intent of the each principle. According to the code's Preamble, the Principles of Ethics ". . . form the underlying moral basis for the Code of Ethics" (American Speech-Language-Hearing Association, 1992b, p. 1). The Rules of Ethics are more specific. The Rules of Ethics give minimum standards of acceptable professional behavior. Following is a discussion of the four major principles of the code.

Principle of Ethics I

> Individuals shall honor their responsibility to hold paramount the welfare of persons they serve professionally. (ASHA, 1992b, p. 1)

Protecting the client's welfare is the primary emphasis of the entire Code of Ethics. One might assume that, of course, concern about a client's welfare is paramount. But, exactly what factors are involved in this?

Preparation

Service providers must be well prepared and be able to perform competently. In training programs, both student clinicians and clinical supervisors must abide by this mandate. Competent service delivery suggests that you are able to perform procedures accurately and effectively. To do this, you often must prepare in advance for each client. Initially, your preparation for clinical practicum involves completion of certain academic courses. You will complete many undergraduate courses related to communicative disorders. You will also complete specific audiology courses. As you advance in your training, you will complete more specialized courses. The specialized course work helps prepare you to work with specific types of hearing disorders or clients with more complex disorders or behaviors. You may not be assigned certain clients until you have completed courses related to their disorders. For example, you may not be scheduled to work with children until you complete a course in pediatric audiology. In addition to the completion of certain courses, your preparation may include reviewing each client's case history, discussing your evaluation or treatment plans with your clinical supervisor, modifying your plans, reviewing and practicing unfamiliar procedures, and setting up and testing equipment in advance. It also may be necessary for you to research information about certain disorders or diseases mentioned in the client's case history.

To abide by the provisions of Principle I, you must not wait until the last minute to get ready for your practicum assignment. Although your clinical supervisor will be available to assist you if you have questions, or if unanticipated problems arise, it is your professional responsibility to be as well-prepared as possible.

Referrals

Within the premise of providing competent service, the code directs that appropriate referrals be made when necessary. If you are unable to provide adequate service for a client, or if additional services are needed, the client must be referred to individuals who are able to provide the necessary services. For example, it might be necessary for you to refer clients with special communication needs (e.g., the deaf or non-English-speaking) to another audiologist when interpreting services are not available at your practicum site. You also might need to make a referral when clients need specialized testing that cannot be performed in your clinical setting. It is important to note that referrals to other audiologists should be made only to those who hold to the established code of ethical standards.

In addition to referrals to other audiologists, it may be necessary to refer clients to other professionals such as speech-language pathologists or otolaryngologists. To make appropriate referrals, you must understand the roles and responsibilities of different professionals. These will be discussed in Chapter 5.

Discrimination

ASHA has outlined a training program for student clinicians that requires them to work with individuals of different ages and a variety of disorders. You will enjoy working with some age groups more than others and like some individuals better than others. You will find some clients challenging and hope you never have to see them again. However, regardless of your personal or philosophical beliefs, you may not discriminate in your delivery of service due to a client's race, sex, age, religion, national origin, or sexual orientation. Discrimination on the basis of any of these factors is prohibited by the ASHA Code of Ethics.

Do not confuse discrimination with specialization. As a practicing audiologist, you may choose to specialize in pediatric audiology. Then, it is not discrimination if you refuse to see adults in your practice. It is also not considered discrimination if you determine, for example, that you are not able to evaluate a non-English-speaking client accurately when an interpreter is not available. However, it would be considered discrimination if, for example, you refused to see any person born in Lima, Peru whether you could provide appropriate services or not. You must make objective clinical judgments. Avoid letting prejudicial beliefs jeopardize your career.

Informed Consent

The Code of Ethics gives guidelines for communication between the client and the clinician. These guidelines serve to ensure that clients are sufficiently informed to make appropriate decisions to pursue, or not to pursue service. Several rules of ethics in Principle 1 address this. In the beginning of your clinical practicum, your clinical supervisor will model how, what, and to what extent clients are informed. As you become more independent in providing clinical service, it is important that you develop an ethical basis for giving information.

Several of the Rules of Ethics give minimal standards for informing clients regarding service. First, the code mandates that clients be told the nature and possible consequences of services provided and products dispensed. You will learn to discuss testing procedures and subsequent results and recommendations with your clients. You also will learn to inform clients fully regarding the type of amplification recommended, including the cost of the hearing aid, warranties, and follow-up services provided.

Second, within the realm of fully informing the client, the code directs that results of services or products cannot be guaranteed. However, appropriate prognostic statements can be made. For example, based on a client's medical history, family history, hearing test results, and hearing aid specifications, you determine that a specific type of hearing aid would most improve the client's hearing. Although your decision is based on reliable data, many variables affect treatment and effective use of amplification. You cannot guarantee that a specific hearing aid, assistive listening device, or other form of intervention will be 100% effective. However, you can provide information based on your data and knowledge of treatment. You can discuss your prognosis and the variables that may affect treatment with your client.

Third, the code states that you may not charge for services not provided or misrepresent services or products. This rule also implies that you accurately communicate with third-party payers, such as insurance companies. You must be ethical in providing and charging for service. You may not guarantee that products can do something they cannot do. If you have a financial interest in a particular product, or business, you should communicate this to your client. You must not make clinical recommendations based on your financial benefit. For example, if you have financial interest in a specific hearing aid, but that particular aid would not be the most effective for your client, you must recommend the most effective aid and not the one from which you would make the most money.

To ensure that services are not misrepresented, university clinics often require clients to sign a statement indicating that they know services are provided by supervised student clinicians. University clinics also may require individuals to sign a written statement verifying their understanding of possible consequences of treatment, plans of treatment, and product warranties and return policies.

If any of your clients are involved in a research project, they must be fully informed of this. Your university and the clinic will have guidelines for protecting human subjects who participate in research studies. Typically, a Human Subjects Protection Committee reviews research proposals and approves their methods and procedures. Your clients have the right to refuse participation in research projects with no consequences. Therefore, before you begin a research project, you should submit a proposal to the Human Subjects Protection Committee of your department, school, or university.

Check to make sure all documents requiring the client's signature for consent for service are signed before you begin working with the client. You may need to discuss the forms with the client to be sure that they understand the meaning of each form.

Treatment Efficacy

The ASHA Code of Ethics prohibits dispensing products or providing services from which a client cannot reasonably be expected to benefit. One might typically interpret this rule as prohibiting audiologists (or others) from ordering more than is needed, but the opposite—not recommending sufficient treatment—also can apply. For example, you may determine that an individual requires binaural amplification, but the funding agency will pay for only one hearing aid. Under the Code of Ethics, if a single hearing aid would not benefit your client, you still must recommended two, regardless of the regulations of the funding agency. Your educational and clinical experience (and that of your clinical supervisor) initially will direct you in determining the most appropriate services for your clients. You will need to determine the correct tests to administer and, based on the results of the tests, the appropriate recommendations to make. You must not recommend tests that you do not think will provide any valuable or relevant information. Nor should you recommend hearing aids or other treatment from which your client would not benefit. Of course, you cannot predict with 100% accuracy what types of habilitative treatment will be most useful for your client. However, you can make clinical choices and recommendations based on your education, clinical data, and supervisory input. Your supervisor will model the correct way to inform clients of results and recommendations.

Confidentiality

The Code of Ethics protects clients' rights to privacy. Rule 1.I of the code states, "Individuals will not reveal, without authorization, any professional or personal information about the person served professionally, unless required by law to do so, or unless doing so is necessary to protect the welfare of the person or of the community" (ASHA, 1992b, p. 1). You will be involved in issues of client confidentiality early in your academic career. As a student observer, you are required to respect and maintain client confidentiality in the same manner as student clinicians, clinical supervisors, and office staff. It is imperative that, throughout your clinical practicum and later professional practice, you understand the importance of upholding client confidentiality.

Clinic sessions are observed on a regular basis at the university clinic by students in the training program. Observations are an integral part of the learning experience for both beginning and advanced students. Because client confidentiality is somewhat compromised by the very nature of the university clinic, observers and student clinicians must respect clients' rights to privacy and adhere to guidelines for protecting client confidentiality.

Flower (1984) described written consent, implied consent, and consent inherent in the private interests of the client. *Written consent* means that the client has signed a written statement giving his or her approval for some clinic activity. Written consent can be used for both informing clients and protecting clients' rights to confidentiality. It is not uncommon to have clients sign consent forms indicating their approval for observations, photographs, videotapes, release of certain information, and service delivery by student clinicians. With few exceptions, written authorization is required before any client information can be released to another agency or professional. This is true of both on- and off-campus practicum sites. It is often the clinic secretary's responsibility to make sure that a written authorization is in the client's folder before releasing written reports. However, you may be involved in initially contacting the client to obtain the authorization. Discuss the procedures for releasing confidential information with your clinic supervisor.

In *implied consent*, no written approval is given, nor is it deemed necessary. When clients seek services at the clinic by completing case histories or other application forms, clients give implicit approval for access to their records by the office staff and other clinic personnel. In this case, it is not necessary for the clinic to obtain written consent from a prospective client for the clinic secretary or other clinic personnel to review the client information. However, all clinic personnel still must protect clients' confidentiality.

There are some instances when information must be released without the permission of the client. These circumstances occur when it is determined that release of the information would benefit the client. Release of information in these instances is acceptable under the condition of consent inherent in the private interests of the client. In cases of suspected child abuse, drug abuse, or medical necessity, it may be necessary for you to release information to outside agencies or other family members. In these types of situations, you first must discuss any communication and release of information with your clinic supervisor.

Your university will have guidelines relating to client confidentiality. These guidelines will include procedures for checking out files, removing information from files, recording information in files, discussing client information with other professionals, and sending copies of reports to other professionals or agencies. Off-campus practicum sites also will have procedures for protecting client confidentiality. You must adhere to the specific guidelines of each on- and off-campus site. The following are some general recommendations for protecting client confidentiality.

1. **Avoid discussing your clients in public areas.** It is natural, and a good learning experience, for you and other student clinicians to discuss clients and clinical activities. However, you must use good judgment regarding where, when, and how much to discuss with other students. Although you may have the best intentions of maintaining your client's confidentiality, conversations can easily be overheard. Even if the

unauthorized listener does not know your client by name, they may have observed you with your client, or they may just get the wrong impression of what your clinical experience was all about. You do not need to be paranoid, just cautious. Do not discuss your client by name, and do not discuss your clients outside of the clinic area. Within the confines of the clinic, do not speak loudly or make fun of your client or something your client did.

2. **Do not discuss your client by name unless necessary.** Obviously, when you discuss your client with your supervisor or during clinic staffing it is necessary and appropriate to discuss your client by name. However, if you are presenting a case history for one of your classes, you can disguise the identity of the client through the use of an alias, initials, or nonspecific references such as "my client."

3. **Give reports, lesson plans, or other written information containing client information directly to your supervisor.** Do not leave material containing confidential client information unattended. Unless you know specifically what client information is considered confidential and what is not, assume that all written reports, test forms, audiograms, and correspondence are confidential.

4. **Do not remove client records from the clinic.** You may have a "working file" of clinical information that you take home. However, this file should not contain clinical documents. Confidential information should not be removed from the clinical facility.

5. **Discuss your client with other professionals agencies only when your client or your supervisor has approved it.** Your supervisor may approve the communication to protect the welfare of the client or the community. It may be necessary for you to telephone other professionals regarding the results of your evaluation or recommendations. Be sure that your client has signed any necessary release forms allowing you to share information with other agencies or individuals. Occasionally it may be necessary to communicate with another agency without the permission of the client. For example, if you suspect that a client may be a victim of child abuse, you will need to report the information to an agency such as child protective services. In this case, you do not need the permission of the child or the parent or guardian. However, you will need to discuss your concerns with your clinical supervisor before taking any action. It is always important to adhere to clinic rules regarding release of client information.

Other rules related to holding client welfare paramount leave little room for interpretation. These rules prohibit managing or evaluating a client through correspondence only, charging for services not provided, and engaging in practice when you have a substance abuse problem or mental or emotional disability that interferes with appropriate service delivery. In addition, although not always related to direct client service, all the Principles of Ethics assist in ensuring the highest quality of service to clients.

Principle of Ethics II

> Individuals shall honor their responsibility to achieve and maintain the highest level of professional competence. (ASHA, 1992b, p. 1)

Principle II discusses several factors related to professional qualifications. As you know, ASHA has defined the minimum qualifications of the profession as those necessary for the Certificate of Clinical Competence (CCC). The code mandates that only individuals holding the Certificate of Clinical Competence, or supervised individuals in the certification process, may provide services in speech-language pathology or audiology. Supervision of candidates in their clinical fellowship year (CFY) and student interns also is restricted to individuals who hold ASHA certification. Services may be provided by individuals only in the area in which they are certified. For example, individuals holding the CCC-A can provide all audiological services they are qualified to provide, and they can screen for speech and language disorders. However, they cannot evaluate and treat speech and language disorders. Also, the code advises that professionals may not provide services they are not competent to perform. For example, an otherwise competent audiologist may not be trained in intraoperative monitoring.

It is impossible to provide competent service when your equipment is in poor working order. Therefore, the code directs that equipment be well maintained and instruments be correctly calibrated. You will learn calibration guidelines and procedures in your course work. As a professional, it will be your responsibility to ensure that these guidelines and procedures are followed.

Continuing education is recommended in the Code of Ethics. Your training as an audiologist does not end when you finish your graduate work, nor does it end when you complete your CFY. As a recent graduate, you will have the fundamental skills on which to build. During your CFY, you will be able to refine these skills, expand your knowledge, and develop your own professional style. Because the profession of audiology is rapidly changing, continuing education and professional development is necessary to maintain a high level of professional competence.

ASHA does not require a certain number of continuing education units or hours for you to maintain your certification, as do some other professional organizations. However, your state's licensing board may require continuing education to maintain your hearing aid dispensing license. For example, in California six units of continuing education credit are required annually.

Principle of Ethics III

Individuals shall honor their responsibility to the public by promoting public understanding of the professions, by supporting the development of services designed to fulfill the unmet needs of the public, and by providing accurate information in all communications involving any aspect of the professions. (ASHA, 1992b, p. 2)

Accurate representation of the profession is an important aspect of provision of clinical services at university training programs. Clients must be fully informed that services are provided by student clinicians. It is unethical for students or professionals to misrepresent their qualifications or training. At the university clinic, clients may be asked to sign a form indicating they understand that services are provided by students. Students often wear identification badges with their names and titles. At off-campus sites, it is equally important for students to identify themselves and explain their status to clients.

Representation of the profession also addresses advertising and marketing. Audiology is becoming a competitive profession. Private practices are growing. The code directs that individuals follow professional standards when advertising. The public should not be misled. All information provided to the public must be accurate.

Principle of Ethics IV

Individuals shall honor their responsibilities to the profession and their relationships with colleagues, students, and members of allied professions. Individuals shall uphold the dignity and autonomy of the professions, maintain harmonious interprofessional and intraprofessional relationships, and accept the professions' self-imposed standards. (ASHA, 1992b, p. 2)

In upholding their professional responsibilities, individuals must be honest. Again, professionals are directed not to misrepresent themselves or perform in any way that is a detriment to the profession. Individuals must provide accurate information to the public and to colleagues. Also, credit must be given for work performed. For example, individuals who have contributed to a paper or presentation must be recognized. You have seen such credit assigned in many of your textbooks and in journal articles. You also must give credit to other students who helped you author a paper or prepare a presentation. In addition, you must make appropriate reference citations in your reports and papers.

Under Principle IV of the Code of Ethics, supervisors are mandated to ensure that individuals under their supervision uphold the Code of Ethics. In clinical practicum, your supervisor will be evaluating not only your educational skill level, but also your professionalism.

If you have reason to believe that an ASHA member has violated the Code of Ethics, the code states that it is your responsibility to inform the Ethical Practice Board of ASHA and fully cooperate in the investigation. As a student clinician, you should first report your concerns to your clinical supervisor. It is expected that soon after you report your concerns that the clinic director and the department chair will be informed and appropriate action taken.

Sections of the Code of Ethics have been highlighted in this chapter. You should read the entire Code of Ethics in Appendix C. Discuss professional issues with your clinic supervisor. If you have any questions about whether a specific behavior falls outside the realm of ethical behavior, talk to your clinic supervisor immediately.

Other Codes and Regulations

Scope of Practice

ASHA has published a scope of practice statement for speech-language pathology and audiology (ASHA, 1990c) and a directory of preferred practice patterns for speech-language pathology and audiology (ASHA, 1993b). These documents outline types of services, the professional performing the service, the expected outcome, clinical indicators, clinical process, any equipment specifications, safety and health precautions, documentation, and related references. The scope of clinical practice in audiology is expanding. As a practicum student, you should be familiar with existing documents addressing scope of practice and preferred patterns of practice. You also should keep current with discussions related to proposed changes in scope and preferred patterns of practice. Such discussion is a topic of journal articles, newsletters, and sessions at professional conferences.

Reporting Suspected Child Abuse

You will encounter many situations in which you will have to make rational and ethical judgments. A case that involves evaluating information and weighing protection of client confidentiality against the protection of the client is suspected child abuse. In most clinical activities, you will assume that all client information is confidential. However, in cases of suspected child abuse, the need to protect the child supersedes the client's right to confidentiality. The specific definition and parameters of child abuse differ from state to state. Generally, child abuse refers to an action or lack of action that endangers a child's,physical or emotional well-being. This may include physical, sexual, or emotional abuse. Neglect also may be included in the definition of child abuse.

If you suspect that a child client of yours is a victim of abuse, you must report your suspicions to your supervisor immediately. Each state has laws and regulations governing the reporting of child abuse. Some states also include reporting of neglect within the same reporting parameters of child abuse. There is no universal standard for reporting information; however, generally the professional who suspects the abuse is responsible for reporting it to the appropriate state agency. States differ in the definition of child abuse, the age range of victims, and the agency to whom information must be reported (Flower, 1984). Child abuse definitions and reporting procedures also may be altered due to legal judgments.

If you are working with a client whom you suspect is a victim of child abuse, do not contact the responsible state agency, but discuss your concerns with your supervisor immediately. Your supervisor can help you evaluate the situation and inform you of your responsibilities in reporting suspected child abuse. Because you will be closely supervised as a student clinician, and because your clients are also your supervisor's clients, you may not be required to be the sole informant. Child abuse is not always easy to identify. Children often acquire bruises, cuts, scrapes, and even broken bones as a result of innocent accidents. It is not necessary to be suspicious of every scratch or bruise, but it is wise to ask the child how the injury occurred. You should be aware of some of the signs of child abuse that Burke (1990) identified:

1. Physical abuse indicators include burns, broken bones, bruises, bites, and cigarette burns.
2. Scratches and bruises located on areas of the body other than shins, elbows, or knees may be more indicative of child abuse than of accidental injury.
3. Bilateral injuries.
4. Inappropriately clothed child. For example, a child who wears long sleeved clothing during hot summer months.
5. Unexplained injuries.
6. Large number of absences from school in the absence of serious illness.
7. Behavioral difficulties, including distrust of adults, listlessness, hostility, depression, self-destructiveness, overly compulsive behavior, or withdrawal.
8. Overly sophisticated in sexual knowledge.
9. Seductive with peers and adults.
10. Dirty, inadequately clothed, malnourished children with unmet dental and medical needs may be victims of neglect.

These are only a few of the *indicators* of child abuse. Again, indicators mean that they suggest something, but do not prove that it exists. You should consider all factors and discuss individual clients with your supervisor before jumping to the conclusion that a client is a victim of child abuse. But you should not rule out or ignore the fact that you may work with children who are victims of abuse, and you are required to take some action in reporting suspected abuse.

Dress Code

Individuals typically are judged on their appearances. The way you look may inspire confidence or distrust. You may more easily establish rapport or quickly turn people off based on your attire and demeanor. The manner in which you dress and even wear your hair may detract or enhance your clinical sessions. Although there is not a common clinical practicum dress code, you must use common sense in your choice of attire. You do not need to purchase expensive clothes. You do need to appear professional. You will want to wear comfortable clothing that is neat and clean. Both male and female students should avoid wearing jeans, sandals, shorts, or provocative clothing. Clinicians must consider modesty and comfort in situations where there is frequent kneeling and bending, such as in school hearing screening.

Different practicum sites have different dress standards. Dress according to the standards at your assigned site. At hospital sites, you may wear casual professional attire and the traditional white lab coat; at a private clinic, you may dress more formally; at some school sites, you may dress less formally, but not unprofessionally. If you are not aware of the appropriate attire at your practicum assignment, ask your supervisor.

Liability Insurance

Because they provide direct clinical services, even student clinicians may be held liable for any inappropriate or negligent service that damages or harms clients. You could also be involved in a frivolous lawsuit with no legal basis. Nonetheless, you could be at financial risk. Therefore, you need professional liability insurance. Professional liability insurance can help protect you against claims of malpractice. Some liability insurance also pays court costs for you.

Your department will have guidelines for obtaining liability insurance. A low-cost insurance policy is available on an annual basis to most students. Some universities pay the insurance as part of your lab fee; others ask students to contract individually with the insurance company. Regardless of the procedures, you should have liability insurance before beginning clinical practicum at any site.

If you encounter a clinical situation in which you are unsure how to proceed, or if you feel that you are unable to provide appropriate service to a particular client, inform your supervisor immediately. To decrease the chance of any appearance of negligence or impropriety, you should be aware of your abilities and limitations. Of course, you will not always be performing services you are familiar with. Part of being a student is learning new information and practicing new ways of doing things. An effective way of avoiding potentially inappropriate professional behavior is to adhere strictly to the ASHA Code of Ethics, comply with all clinic procedures, and follow current standards of practice as recommended in ASHA Position Statements and Guidelines, Scope of Practice, and Preferred Practice Patterns.

Health and Safety Precautions

There are precautions you will want to take to protect your own safety and health and that of your clients. Certain health regulations must be followed when you work closely with many different people. These regulations are fairly universal and provide protection from variouscommunicable diseases. Safety precautions also are fairly standard. However, both health and safety regulations may vary somewhat from site to site. Therefore, find out the regulations of your clinical assignment and follow them. The following are some general health precautions.

1. **Get a rubella vaccination.** You only need to be vaccinated against rubella once; however, it is a an important vaccination. Rubella, often called German measles, can cause several serious complications to the developing fetus, including death. Although this viral disease is often accompanied by a fever and a rash, children who have rubella usually do not experience severe complications. The serious danger is to the unborn child (Benenson, 1990).

2. **Get a mumps vaccination.** Mumps is a viral infection accompanied by fever and tenderness and swelling of the salivary glands. Mumps vaccinations are recommended for male health care providers because of the incidence of testicular mumps in the male population. There is no conclusive evidence that mumps during pregnancy causes birth defects. However, it is a preventable disease and its incidence in the United States increased in 1986 and 1987 (Benenson, 1990.)

3. **Have a Tuberculin skin test** (PPD - Purified Protein Derivative). You may be required to have an annual Tuberculin test (TB test) or the test may be required less frequently. Be sure to adhere to your clinic's guidelines regarding the frequency of this test. Tuberculosis often goes unrecognized in its initial stage and the incidence of TB in the United States is on the increase. There is no vaccination against TB, but regular testing will decrease the chances of serious effects. If untreated, tuberculosis can cause serious complications, including death (Benenson, 1990).

4. **Use gloves.** Wear latex gloves when performing any invasive procedure or during any contact with blood or bodily fluids with visible blood (ASHA Committee on Quality Assurance, 1990). Also, if you are wearing gloves to protect the client against infection, when wearing gloves do not touch your pencil, the table, the chair, or other objects after you have put on the gloves.

5. **Wash your hands before and after working with a client.** You have probably seen the sign in bathrooms, "Hand washing is one of the best ways to prevent the spread of disease." Take this statement seriously.

6. **Disinfect or sterilize equipment.** Your practicum site will have specific regulations concerning sterilization and disinfection of equipment. ASHA suggests that disinfection can be performed using 1:100 solution of household bleach (sodium hypochlorite) to water, or you may use commercial disinfectant (ASHA Committee on Quality

Assurance, 1990). Be aware that hepatitis requires exposure to a 1:10 solution of household bleach for 14 hours before it is killed. Many audiology clinics use reusable probe tips for immittance testing and reusable speculums for otoscopy. These must be disinfected prior to use with another client. They should be retrieved from containers with tweezers and handled in tissue to ensure sanitary handling of devices to be inserted into the client's ear.

7. **Use disposable materials.** Rather than worrying about disinfecting equipment, it is preferable to use disposable materials whenever possible.

8. **If you are ill, cancel your clinical appointments.** You know how you feel when you are working with a client who is sneezing and coughing. You wish they had stayed home because you know you probably will get whatever they have. Well, the client feels the same way about you. If you are ill, follow your clinic protocol for rescheduling clients.

9. **Be knowledgeable about communicable diseases.** There are many diseases the audiologist must be aware of. The degree of concern regarding certain diseases may vary depending on the population you are working with. However, the best way to prevent the spread of disease is to be educated about it, not to ignore the existence of communicable diseases or be fearful of them. One disease that we are still learning more about is Acquired Immune Deficiency Syndrome (AIDS). AIDS and HIV infection are a major health concern (ASHA Committee on Quality Assurance, 1989; ASHA Committee on Quality Assurance, 1990; McMillan & Willette, 1988). There is presently no known cure for AIDS, which ultimately results in death. AIDS infection is not spread by normal social contact. It is believed to be transmitted by sexual exposure or exposure to blood or tissues (Benenson, 1990).

Knowing and understanding the variety of health precautions used at each of your practicum sites may require some research on your part. However, a few safety precautions are universal and based on common sense. The following is a list of some safety precautions.

1. **Make sure the waiting and clinic areas are orderly and clean.**

2. **Do not leave children unattended in the clinic.** Unattended children can get into all sorts of trouble. They can swallow small pieces of equipment, stick their fingers (or other objects) into electrical outlets, get lost, and take a fall. They can get into almost any kind of trouble you can imagine.

3. **Do not let children stand on tables or chairs.** If you need a child to stand on a table or chair for some reason, always hold him or her with at least one hand.

4. Do not give children food without first checking with the parent. There probably will be few times when you will be involved in giving a child food. However, if you must give a child food, first check with the parent. The child may have food allergies, swallowing difficulties, a restricted diet, or a parent averse to the child having the food. This caution applies to edible reinforcers you may select for your child client.

5. If clients who are in wheelchairs do not automatically lock their brakes, advise them to do so. If the client is unable to lock his or her own wheelchair brakes, you may lock them.

6. Before pushing a client who is in a wheelchair, make sure the client's feet are in the footrest and the client signals you to proceed. If the client does not use footrests, make sure the client's feet are off the ground before you begin pushing his or her chair.

7. Do not allow smoking in the clinic.

8. Do not leave hearing aid batteries out where young children may ingest them. They are toxic.

As you can now see, there are many codes, regulations, and precautions that you must know and follow. Many of these regulations must be memorized, others are common sense things you do already. Being a competent audiologist involves more than being able to administer and interpret test results or dispense hearing aids. You also must respect and protect your clients' welfare—and respect and protect yourself.

This chapter has discussed a few of the ways in which you can protect your client and yourself. Many other situations will arise when you will have to make decisions based on ethical, safety, or health considerations. As a student clinician, you have your supervisor to help you make those clinical decisions. As a professional audiologist, you will have your experience, your colleagues, ASHA, and your state licensing board to help you make clinically appropriate judgments.

4

The Supervisor and the Student Clinician

A fundamental aspect of the practicum experience is the interaction between the student clinician and the clinical supervisor. Each individual has a defined role to play in the provision of effective service and in the education of the student clinician. These roles are defined by ASHA guidelines on training and supervision, by university and department policies, by area demographics, and by the personalities of the supervisor and student clinician.

First semester practicum students may be anxious about their performance. Administering a procedure for the first time on a "real" client, someone other than a friend or classmate, may cause preperformance anxiety. These feelings are common to most new clinicians. They are so common in other fields of endeavor that our culture has special names for them. New public speakers experience stage fright. Beginning musicians and stage performers experience preperformance jitters. Athletes experience pregame jitters. It is normal, and new students in practicum are expected to experience some preperformance anxiety.

When it is not excessive, preperformance anxiety most often has beneficial effects. One benefit is thorough preparation. To maintain as much control as possible, the student prepares thoroughly for the experience. Another benefit is heightened alertness. Adrenaline flow increases before the actual client contact and the student is in a heightened state of awareness. In such a state, the student is less likely to commit errors. Once the session begins in earnest, preperformance anxiety passes and the student settles into a comfortable routine. At this point, the student may feel overprepared for the experience.

Students perform better when they concentrate on the person receiving their services and, if they are able, forget about how they are performing. If your goal is to communicate instructions in a friendly, clear, and concise manner to a person, rather than to impress your supervisor with your ability to relate, you will do much better.

The Role of the Clinical Supervisor

The clinical supervisor is responsible for training the student clinician while ensuring quality clinical services. The supervisor must meet the educational needs of the student without sacrificing service to the client. To do this, clinical supervisors should be aware of students' academic backgrounds, strengths and weaknesses, the clinical needs of clients, and their own strengths and weaknesses as supervisors. In addition to their primary role of training students in clinical practicum, clinical supervisors often have other responsibilities. For example, at the university clinic, supervisors may also teach academic courses, serve on university committees, function as administrators, or be involved in research projects. In private clinics, supervisors may be involved in such activities as administration, service marketing, and billing and other business operations.

Although many universities have staff who provide only clinical supervision, many other universities and off-campus sites employ supervisors who have duties in addition to those of training interns. While it is imperative for supervisors to understand the strengths and weaknesses of student clinicians, it may be equally important for student clinicians to understand what supervisors can and cannot do and the other responsibilities and obligations supervisors may have. A clear understanding of roles and expectations of both parties helps avoid misunderstandings and unmet needs.

What to Expect from Your Clinical Supervisor

To the student, of course, the supervisor's main responsibility is clinical teaching and supervision. Your clinical supervisor will guide you and assist in your learning in many different ways. Your supervisor may give direct instruction, help you in problem solving and case analysis, guide you in self-evaluation, model specific behaviors or techniques, or refer you to sources for independent study. Various ASHA regulations and guidelines on supervision will influence your supervisor's actions. There are several articles and books on the supervisory process. ASHA periodically publishes information to update or clarify information related to clinical supervision. In 1985, the ASHA Committee on Supervision published a position statement on the tasks of clinical supervision in speech-language pathology and audiology. This position statement did not reiterate the regulations concerning the amount and type of supervision but, instead, described specific tasks, competencies, and supervisor preparation leading to effective clinical supervision. The tasks outlined in the ASHA position statement have been used to outline some of the behaviors you can expect from your clinical supervisor (ASHA Committee on Supervision, 1985). Your clinical supervisor will do the following.

1. **Facilitate effective communication.** The communication process is two-sided. Both the student clinician and the supervisor must be willing participants in the development and maintenance of effective communication. Otherwise, no matter how clearly one individual expresses suggestions, ideas, or questions, the other may not accurately receive or interpret the information. It is imperative that a good communication system be developed between supervisors and student clinicians. This will create a better learning environment and assist in more effective service delivery. To help establish a predictable method of communication, supervisors may schedule regular clinic meeting times, individual conference times, periodic evaluation sessions, or written feedback. In addition to regularly scheduled meetings, many supervisors may be available before, after, and during clinic sessions and during regular office hours.

In discussing clinical plans or reviewing a clinic session with you, supervisors may attempt to gain an understanding of your level of comprehension or clarify information by asking you questions, requiring you to describe events in measurable terms, or asking you to problem-solve orally something that happened in your clinic session. Communication from your supervisor should be supportive. However, it may not always be positive. Hopefully, your supervisor will have the skills necessary to give you informative feedback and assist you in developing your own communication and clinical skills without insulting you. You should not feel humiliated by your supervisor. If you do, you should discuss your feelings with your supervisor and, if this does not help, possibly with your department chairperson or clinic director. On the other hand, when you receive praise after you have performed well, you will want to know more than that you did a "good job." Your supervisor will give you specific information. For example, "Good, you were able to work through the child's behavior problem, because you knew the equipment and test better and administered the test 50% faster than last time." Remember, it is your supervisor's job to point out both your strengths and your weaknesses and to help you improve. However, supervisors know only what they can observe. You may have questions or concerns your supervisor is not aware of. Do not hesitate to ask questions or discuss ideas with your supervisor. Your active involvement in communications with your supervisor will enhance your working relationship.

Supervision styles vary greatly. There are probably as many styles of supervision as there are supervisors. Some supervisors demonstrate procedures on the first person seen and then watch the student clinician on subsequent contacts, offering suggestions and encouragement as needed. Other supervisors concentrate on areas in which the student could improve and make suggestions during the process. Still other supervisors take notes and discuss the student's strengths and weakness after the activity is concluded. Many supervisors do a combination of these things. Most supervisors are considerate and helpful. Regardless of supervision style, the supervisor will be physically available on site.

2. **Describe practicum requirements.** To develop effective communication and to facilitate a good learning experience, your clinical supervisor will give you specific information regarding the requirements of your clinical practicum assignment. Your supervisor may give you an overview of the semester and then discuss specific requirements. Timelines for beginning and ending the term will be given, as well as timelines for individual clinic appointments. For example, you may begin your clinic assignment on September 1 and complete the assignment on December 15. You may be required to see clients 1 day per week. Clients may be scheduled every hour, every 2 hours, or every half hour, or appointments may vary depending on the client's problem. Your supervisor will explain how you find out your daily clinic schedule, who your clients are, and when you meet with the supervisor to discuss clinic

plans. Your supervisor also will explain reporting requirements, such as notations in the clients' charts, recording information on test protocols, writing evaluation reports, and acknowledging referrals from outside sources. Your supervisor will outline the grading and performance standards for your clinical practicum. Generally, first semester students will be expected to perform less independently than second semester students, second semester students less independently than third semester students, and so on. Your supervisor also will describe how, and when, you will receive evaluations. There will be minimum requirements you must meet to be able to provide clinical services. These may include overt behaviors such as regular attendance at clinic meetings, punctuality, advance preparation for clinic meetings and appointments (e.g., reading the client's chart in advance), submission of reports on a timely basis, and adequate operation of equipment. Other, less tangible behaviors you may be evaluated on include your professionalism, skill in establishing a working relationship with the clients, and problem-solving skills.

Besides giving you feedback on your performance, your supervisor may discuss future clinical practicum possibilities with you. Your supervisor may suggest assignments he or she thinks would supplement and enhance your training as an audiologist, as well as discuss issues related to meeting ASHA and the university's practicum requirements. Most importantly, your clinic supervisor will be available to answer your questions about clinical practicum. If your supervisor does not have the answer to your questions, he or she will find the answers or refer you to someone who can answer them. To obtain information specific to ASHA requirements, NSSLHA members can phone ASHA's toll-free number (1-800-638-6868). Remember, ASHA requirements are minimum requirements, and your university may have additional standards.

3. **Provide ongoing evaluation of your clinical performance.** Although your clinical supervisor probably will provide you with a formal midterm and final evaluation of your clinical performance, you will want and need more immediate information concerning your strengths and weaknesses. It would do you little good to find out at the time of your final evaluation that throughout the semester you had not performed a certain task correctly. Therefore, clinical supervisors provide feedback throughout the semester. Informative feedback may be provided in written or verbal form. Some supervisors use a formal daily evaluation method. For example, you may receive a grade or points for each of your clinic sessions. At the end of the day your supervisor would provide you with a summary of your performance and a corresponding grade for the day. Other supervisors provide less formal written feedback in the form of short notes. Many supervisors

regularly provide verbal feedback. Your supervisor may give instructional and encouraging feedback while you are working with a client or immediately after the session. You also may be scheduled to meet with your supervisor on a regular basis to discuss specific clients as well as your clinical performance.

Feedback is essential to your learning experience. However, after receiving some initial feedback, you will want and need to develop self-analysis skills. In the beginning, you will not have the experience and knowledge to evaluate your own performance fully or that of your clients. Therefore, you will need to rely on your supervisor for assistance. Different supervisors provide different amounts of feedback. One semester you may work with a supervisor who provides you with daily written and verbal feedback. The next semester you may work with a supervisor who gives you feedback only when you ask questions. Most supervisors try to balance the amount of feedback they give with the amount of self-analysis they wish you to develop. The supervisor who provides little feedback may be trying to assist you in developing problem-solving skills. If you feel you are getting too little feedback or, conversely, not being allowed to solve problems on your own, discuss your concerns with your clinical supervisor.

4. **Assist in planning and organizing clinic sessions.** Before meeting with a client you need to review the client's chart and case history to determine which tests and procedures will be most appropriate to use with the client. For example, if you are scheduled to evaluate a developmentally delayed child, your goals for the first session may be to establish rapport, condition the child to wear the earphones, and condition the child to respond consistently to a test tone. You probably will meet with your supervisor on a regular basis to review the plans for each of your clients. Your supervisor may instruct you to review the chart, plan and organize your session, and prepare to present your plan at a weekly clinic meeting. Sometimes, you may not know who your client will be until just a few minutes before the session. In these cases, you usually will have time to discuss your plan briefly with your supervisor before the session. Supervisors may have a specific format for student clinicians to follow for each clinic session. For example, your supervisor may instruct you to first interview the client, then perform a pure-tone audiometric evaluation, followed by immittance audiometry. Organization of clinical sessions and test procedures are discussed in Parts II, III, and IV.

5. **Help develop diagnostic skills.** Your clinical supervisor will observe at least half of each of your diagnostic sessions. If you are a beginning student clinician, are assigned a complex case, or are at an off-

campus site, your supervisor may observe more than 50% of the session. Your supervisor may help you develop your diagnostic skills by giving you suggestions and pointing out information while you are working with your client. Your supervisor also may discuss evaluation information before and after clinical sessions. Your supervisor may suggest a certain sequence for administering tests, techniques for eliciting certain behaviors, methods for testing difficult clients, and so on. Observation of the evaluation session helps ensure quality service delivery, but also allows direct instruction for the student clinician. Your supervisor is not observing just to grade you, but to help you develop effective clinical skills. Your supervisor will help you learn which tests are the most appropriate for certain clients, how to administer different tests, how to evaluate your client's behavior and your own behavior in the clinical setting, and how to interpret test information and apply that information to individual clients.

6. **Demonstrate different clinical techniques and procedures.** Before beginning your clinical practicum, you will have studied many clinical techniques and procedures. Observing the implementation of these techniques and procedures is an essential part of learning. Textbooks are not able to cover every clinical situation. Also, you may interpret written instructions differently than they were intended, or your supervisor may use some shortcuts, or slightly different procedures than those described in your text. If you have difficulty understanding a certain procedure, if your supervisor wants to illustrate an instruction better, or if your supervisor wants to teach you a new procedure, he or she may model the procedure. If you have trouble understanding an instruction, ask your supervisor to demonstrate it for you.

7. **Help you learn different intervention options and develop management skills.** In your academic course work, you will study current research and learn basic hearing management strategies. In clinical practicum, you will learn to apply the research information and assessment and management strategies to individual clients. Your supervisor will help you identify the subtleties imperative for successful intervention. Your supervisor may specify a sequence for you to follow in assessing hearing problems and providing habilitative services, or your supervisor may allow you to develop a new sequence. An important aspect of management is the ability to document changes in your client's behavior. Your supervisor will assist you in learning to use measurable descriptors. For example, you should document the changes (improvement) in speech reception in clients for whom you have prescribed hearing aids. In aural rehabilitation, you should develop both short- and long-term goals for your clients. When you assess hearing, you should

make appropriate prognostic statements that apply to different management strategies or no strategies. It is important to be able to identify and analyze your own clinical behaviors.

8. **Explain documentation and record keeping requirements.** Each of your practicum sites will have different documentation and record keeping requirements. Some sites require extensive documentation of each appointment, including a written report. Other sites require only brief handwritten notes on the final recommendations or outcome of the session. Generally, there will be some similarities across settings. For example, most sites will require you to file a copy of the client's audiogram in the client's folder, maintain the clients' charts in a neat and orderly manner, and protect client confidentiality. Your supervisor will discuss the requirements, policies, and procedures at your practicum site. If you do not understand the rationale for a certain requirement, do not ignore the requirement, assuming that it is frivolous or a waste of time. Ask your supervisor to explain the rationale for the policy or procedure. Often, it is based on accreditation standards or third-party reimbursement requirements.

9. **Facilitate independence and self-evaluation.** Effective supervision allows student clinicians progressively greater degrees of independence while helping them learn to evaluate their own clinical sessions. Initially, your clinical supervisor will provide direct and frequent supervision, identifying specific behaviors you need to change, tasks you need to learn and clinical strengths you need to continue to emphasize. As you gain clinical experience, your clinical supervisor will allow you more independence in making clinical decisions and ask you to begin evaluating different aspects of your clinical sessions. You will be expected to describe the strengths and weaknesses of your session. Your supervisor may schedule regular formal conferences when you will be asked to give a summary and analysis of your clinical sessions, or your supervisor may talk with you on a less formal basis during and following clinical sessions. Occasionally, you may feel that your supervisor is not giving you a direct answer to your questions. Try not to be offended by this. Your supervisor may judge that you can research the question and obtain the answer with supervisory assistance.

10. **Help develop oral and written reporting skills.** As an audiologist, you will be required to write many reports and regularly discuss assessment results and clinical recommendations with clients and other professionals. As a student clinician, your clinical supervisor will help you develop both oral and written reporting skills by requiring you to perform these tasks and giving you feedback on your work. Your supervisor will give you guidelines to follow, although you will eventually develop your own unique style.

The reporting requirements at each practicum site will vary. At some sites you may write reports daily. At other sites, you may do very little writing, but frequently report information orally. Regardless of the format requirements at each site, you need to report information in a clear, concise, and accurate manner. In both written and verbal reports, you should use correct grammar and vocabulary. Spelling and punctuation must be accurate in written reports. If you are assigned to a setting where a secretary or data transcriber writes your reports, your supervisor will help you learn to give adequate and appropriate information to help those individuals correctly write your report.

11. **Provide, or refer you to, current resources.** Although you will have textbooks containing much basic information, technology is rapidly supplying the profession of audiology with new information and equipment. Your supervisor will help you keep up with current equipment, procedures, and theories by giving you information or referring you to other sources where you can obtain the information. Because of the progressive changes in audiology, you need to develop a method of routinely updating your clinical information. ASHA, AAA, and the other professional organizations encourage their members to do this through continuing education programs. Many state licensure laws require registration of continuing education units.

12. **Exhibit and require professionalism.** There are many aspects to being a professional. Your supervisor will model the behavior he or she expects from you and may give you guidelines for specific behaviors. For example, different sites may have different dress codes. Certain sites will have specific guidelines for protecting client confidentiality. Other sites may determine that protection of client confidentiality is inherent in the setting and written guidelines are not necessary. Regardless of the formality or informality of your practicum site, you will always be required to know and uphold the ASHA Code of Ethics. The code outlines minimal standards for professional behavior. Periodically, review the code to ensure that you are familiar with its principles.

13. **Assess your clinical performance.** In addition to assisting you with clinical service delivery and helping you develop your clinical skills, your supervisor must evaluate your performance. Your supervisor will discuss your strengths and weaknesses, may ask you to describe your strengths and weaknesses, and may instruct you to develop some personal objectives to work on. Your supervisor may give you informal feedback throughout the semester as well as more formal feedback during a midterm or final evaluative conference. Your evaluation is usually translated into a letter grade.

14. **Act as your mentor.** Your supervisor will help guide you through your clinical practicum assignment and challenge you to give

your optimal performance. Your supervisor will help you obtain the experiences necessary to meet your university's and ASHA's clinical requirements. Your supervisor may also help direct you to other practicum assignments that could give you experience in areas you are interested in pursuing or in areas you need to improve.

The Off-Campus Clinical Supervisor

During your assignment at an on-campus audiology clinic, you will work with supervisors who are familiar with the university's academic and clinical requirements. These supervisors may be full- or part-time members of the university community. Often, off-campus supervision is provided by professionals employed at the off-campus practicum site. These professionals may or may not be familiar with your training program and its requirements. Your off-campus supervisor may behave differently and have different expectations than did your on-campus supervisors.

Probably, your off-campus supervisor will perform many of the same duties of your on-campus supervisor. Your supervisor will expect you to perform professionally, manage clients effectively, and work diligently to increase your abilities. Your off-campus supervisor will give you feedback regarding your performance, supervise your clinical sessions, and assist you in gaining a variety of experiences in the setting.

Your off-campus supervisor may or may not provide the amount of supervision you are familiar with; however, the supervisor will minimally adhere to ASHA's guidelines on supervision. In fact, at least initially, off-campus supervisors may provide 100% supervision because each site may have only one student clinician, the supervisors are not familiar with the student's training, and third-party reimbursement or client public relations require the presence of a licensed audiologist during delivery of services.

Your introduction to clinical practicum begins at the on-campus clinic. When you begin off-campus practicum assignments, you are expected to be able to perform fairly independently. Your off-campus supervisor will expect you to perform many routines without being given specific instructions. For example, you may be told to write a report according to the specific format of the site. Your off-campus supervisor may expect you to look at previous reports or develop your own report. In essence, you will be expected to behave as a professional.

An off-campus supervisor who does not know you or your background fully may assign you clients with whom you do not feel competent to work. Be sure to discuss your concerns with your supervisor. Let your supervisor know your background. Do not pretend you have more experience than you do. Your experience will be apparent when you begin working with clients.

Your off-campus supervisor's role is to help you learn. If you feel you are not gaining the experience or getting the support you need, discuss your concerns with the off-campus supervisor. If concerns persist, discuss them with you advisor on the campus.

The Responsibilities of Student Clinicians

Student clinicians have many responsibilities. While balancing personal obligations, you must fulfill requirements of academic courses and complete clinical practicum duties. As part of your clinical practicum, you must learn both the clinical and interpersonal skills necessary to evaluate, treat, and counsel clients and their families effectively and accurately. As you know, during the initial stages of your practicum training, your supervisor will provide more direct supervision and instruction. As you gain more experience and confidence, your supervisor will expect you to perform more independently.

Each training program has certain unique requirements. However, some standards are typical of most programs. To fulfill your clinical practicum assignments successfully you must do the following:

1. **Know your scope of practice and preferred practice patterns.** In all of your practicum placements, you must be aware of what may be expected of you clinically. Especially as a beginning clinician, you are not expected to be proficient in all areas. You are, however, expected to be familiar with procedures and to know when to apply them. You also are expected to complete basic procedures in a competent manner. Practicum develops timeliness. Practicum develops confidence. Practicum provides experience. Practicum is not a setting for remedial learning.

2. **Use appropriate audiologic diagnostic instruments, tests, or assessment procedures.** Ensure that each evaluation is comprehensive, valid, reliable, and nonbiased. Closely adhere to the test administration guidelines. Follow standard practices for choosing tests and interpreting them.

3. **Know ASHA's Code of Ethics and adhere to its principles.** In all of your assignments as a student clinician, you must comply with ASHA's Code of Ethics. You do not want to jeopardize your future as an audiologist by violating the Code of Ethics. Each of your practicum

settings will present different ethical questions that require an analysis or interpretation of ASHA's Code of Ethics. If you are familiar with the code and its intent, you will be more confident in your behavior or response to certain ethical situations. Refer to Chapter 3 for more detailed information about ASHA's Code of Ethics.

4. **Comply with the policies and procedures of your training program.** Your training program will have many policies and procedures you will have to learn and follow. These may relate to such things as registering for practicum courses, fulfilling health requirements, or submitting reports. Some of these procedures may seem frivolous to you; however, there is a reason for each procedure. Many were developed to avoid a problem or as a consequence of a previous problem. If your training program does not have a procedural handbook, typically the clinic secretary or your clinic supervisor will inform you of the policies and procedures you must follow.

5. **Know and follow the policies and procedures at each of your practicum sites.** In addition to following the policies and procedures of your training program, you must also adhere to the policies and procedures of each of your off-campus assignments. Policies and procedures at off-campus practicum sites may supplement or differ from those of the on-campus clinic, but should not conflict with those of your training program. For example, you will need to follow the training program's procedures for registering for your off-campus clinical practicum, but you will follow the off-campus site's guidelines for report writing.

6. **Respect and maintain the confidentiality of each of your clients.** The topic of client confidentiality is a recurring theme in this book and in your clinical assignments. It is a fundamental right of your clients. Just as you would not want your physician to discuss your health with other people, your clients do not want you to discuss their hearing problems with other people. You also will learn information about clients' families, economic status, and other personal information that must be kept confidential. Follow your practicum site's guidelines regarding the release of client information to outside agencies or other professionals.

7. **Respect each of your clients' cultural and personal beliefs.** To work effectively with clients, you must establish rapport with your client and build his or her trust in you as an expert. To accomplish this, you should learn to respect your client and his or her cultural, ethnic, and social background. Clients who are treated as individuals of worth are likely to trust you and cooperate with you. However, on some occasions, you may have a client whose cultural or personal beliefs conflict with your recommendations. For example, in some

cultures hearing impairment in old age is viewed as a natural process not to be interfered with by hearing aids. To understand why a client is reluctant to accept your recommendation, you need to appreciate such cultural beliefs. You may have to provide additional counseling for some families to educate certain individuals regarding the importance of hearing management. On some occasions, you may realize that your client's cultural or personal beliefs preclude what you consider optimal treatment and have to work within the parameters of that person's belief system.

8. **Be on time and well-prepared for each clinical session.** Prepare, as much as possible, all materials and equipment in advance. Make sure that all necessary equipment is available and operating correctly. Complete all calibration and hearing checks according to your clinic's and ANSI standards. Always be on site 15 to 30 minutes prior to seeing your first client. Do not hold clients longer than their scheduled times. A clinic schedule backed up early in the day is stressful to clients, clinicians, and supervisors alike.

9. **Screen your clients' speech and language performance.** Your practicum site may have formal speech and language screening procedures, such as asking clients to read a standard passage, or you may evaluate your clients' conversational speech. You will screen fluency, articulation, language, and voice. If you determine the possible presence of a speech or language disorders, refer clients to speech-language pathologists for additional testing.

10. **Plan and implement management programs.** Develop management programs that are appropriate to your client's hearing impairment and communication needs assessment. Ensure that the procedures are documented and the results of your intervention are measurable. See Part IV for more specific and detailed information on audiologic management.

11. **Promptly complete and submit all written assignments.** You will have different writing requirements at different practicum sites. Some of your practicum sites will require typewritten reports for each appointment. Others may require only handwritten documentation of the results in the clients' folders. Some sites may require a combination of typewritten reports and handwritten progress notes. Your clinical supervisor will instruct you regarding reporting procedures at your site. Your supervisor also will give you deadlines and timelines for completing reports. If you have any questions about the due date of a report, check with your clinical supervisor.

12. **Maintain accurate clinical records.** Clinical records should be comprehensive, but concise. You will have only a short time in which to note clients' histories, evaluation results, recommendations,

intervention strategies, and results of intervention. A chronological log of clinical activity allows you to retrieve and evaluate your client's services quickly. Sign all test protocols, audiograms, and reports and file them in chronological order. Ensure that your clients' files are kept in an orderly fashion so that you can quickly retrieve important information. Follow your practicum site's guidelines regarding documentation of billing information. Refer to Chapter 5 for more detailed information on record keeping requirements.

13. **Integrate academic course work information into your clinical practicum assignments.** You will learn much of the information necessary for your clinical practicum in your academic courses. Try not to separate the two learning experiences. Applying the information studied in your academic courses to your practicum experiences makes the academic information more relevant and the practicum experiences easier.

14. **Independently gather additional information to enhance your learning.** If you do not know an answer, or a certain procedure, attempt to find the answer independently by researching journals, texts, or test manuals. If your problem remains unsolved, ask your clinic supervisor for help. For several reasons, it is important to learn to solve problems on your own. Researching information usually makes the information more meaningful. Also, in the process, you usually acquire additional information. Finally, as a professional, you may not have associates to assist you in problem solving. You will have to find the answers by yourself to provide effective service.

15. **Ask questions.** This statement may appear contradictory to statement 14; but, actually, it is complimentary. You should learn to research information independently. However, you should also ask questions when you need assistance. You should not risk the quality of service delivery or the audiological needs of your client. Do not work with a client if you are unsure of your ability to do so. Your supervisor will not always know when you need assistance, so you must take the responsibility to ask for needed assistance. You also may want to ask questions regarding the rationale for certain procedures or to gain information about other issues. Remember, one of your supervisor's roles is to help you learn.

16. **Learn to analyze clinical sessions independently.** There are many components to each clinical session. Some of the components involve your behavior, some involve your client's behavior, and others involve assessment or intervention strategies. To work independently, you should learn to analyze all the aspects of a clinical session. Initially, your clinical supervisor will help you evaluate your sessions by giving

you feedback regarding your performance and suggestions on how to improve your service delivery. As you progress in your clinical training, you will learn to analyze the strengths and weaknesses of your clinical skills and each clinical session. You also will learn to apply some of the strategies you use to evaluate your clients' behaviors to your own behaviors. Your supervisor will help you develop self-evaluation and self-analysis skills.

17. **Attend regularly and promptly.** To establish your reputation as a reliable clinician and not disrupt client services, you should attend all scheduled clinical sessions punctually. Each clinical site will have specific procedures to follow if you are ill or have a personal emergency that precludes your clinic attendance. You may not cancel clinical appointments for activities such as studying for exams, taking a vacation, or extending work hours. Your clinical practicum is a professional commitment, and it should receive your highest priority.

18. **Behave in a professional manner.** Although you are still a student, many professional demands are placed on you which you must meet, often on a daily basis. It is sometimes difficult to perform in some situations as a student, and in others as a professional. However, the more you view yourself as a professional, as both a student and a clinician, the easier it will be for you to fulfill your responsibilities in your training program. Certain behaviors give the impression of professionalism, including having knowledge of the clients' disorders, being well prepared and organized for all assignments, being punctual, dressing neatly, and exhibiting respect for yourself, the clinical staff, and your clients.

19. **Keep a log of the clinical clock hours you earn.** Follow your university's established procedures and forms to record the clinical clock hours you earn during your practicum assignments. You probably will be required to maintain both a daily and a semester log of your hours. Periodically, calculate your total hours to ensure you are obtaining hours in the different categories required for ASHA certification, state licensure, and graduation from your university. Although it is the university's responsibility to make sure opportunities are available for you to gain a variety of experiences and earn the necessary clinical clock hours, it is your responsibility to ensure that you take advantage of those opportunities and earn needed clock hours. Refer to Chapter 1 for a detailed discussion of the activities that can be included as clinical clock hours under ASHA guidelines.

20. **Regularly communicate with your clinical supervisor.** Early in your training program you probably will discover that each of your supervisors has a different supervisory style. Some supervisors

will communicate frequently with you on a formal or informal basis. Others may assume that, if you have questions or comments, you will express them without prompts or invitation from the supervisor. It is important to maintain communication with your supervisor, regardless of your practicum site or your supervisor's style of communication. In some cases, you may need to be assertive in asking questions or expressing opinions. In other cases, your supervisor may seek you out on a regular basis to give you opportunities to discuss issues and ask questions. In all cases, you should work cooperatively with your supervisor. Let your supervisor know both the positives and negatives of the practicum experience. Remember, communication is a two-way process.

Your practicum experience will be more rewarding if you know what you can expect from your supervisor and what is expected of you. The description given in this chapter applies to most situations. However, if you have special needs and questions, always talk to your clinical supervisor.

5
Working with Clients

As a student audiologist, you will learn about normal and disordered hearing in your academic courses. In your clinical practicum, you will learn the professional skills of assessment and management of hearing and its disorders. These skills also include interpersonal skills and general procedures for working with clients and other skills such as client scheduling, report writing, record keeping, working with client's families, and working collaboratively with other professionals.

Scheduling Clients

The first step in offering clinical services is to make clinical appointments. The clinic secretary probably will be responsible for making the initial appointment. Always make telephone contact with the client the day before the appointment. Introduce yourself, clarify any case history information, and inform the client that you look forward to meeting him or her. You or the secretary may be responsible for scheduling follow-up appointments. Regardless of who is responsible for initial and follow-up scheduling, it is your responsibility to ensure your client is scheduled for a follow-up appointment. Your clinic schedule and the clients' appointments will be influenced by some of the following variables:

1. **The student clinician's schedule.** Your classes, outside work, family obligations, and so on will influence your clinic schedule.

2. **The availability of clinical supervisors.** As you know, in some settings your clinical supervisors have responsibilities in addition to clinical supervision. For example, at the university clinic, clinical supervisors may also be responsible for teaching courses, advising students, and working on committees.

3. **The student clinician's previous clinical experience.** After you have had a few semesters of clinical practicum experience, you will be able to provide audiological services more efficiently than first semester student clinicians who are not as familiar with equipment or clinic procedures. Therefore, more advanced student clinicians may be given an hour to perform a complete audiological examination, whereas beginning student clinicians may be allowed 2 hours to perform the same services.

4. **The types of clients and convenience of appointments.** At a clinic that provides services primarily for elderly individuals who are retired, the majority of your appointments will be scheduled during the regular 8:00 A.M. to 5:00 P.M. work day. If your site serves many people who work, your appointments may extend past 5:00 P.M., begin before 8:00 A.M., or include a Saturday. If the clinic sees a large number of school-age children, many of your appointments may be scheduled after 3:00 P.M. when the school day ends.

5. **The type and frequency of services needed.** Your clients' needs will also dictate the length of the appointment. Complete audiological assessments may be scheduled hourly. Follow-up appointments may be scheduled for 15-30 minute intervals. It is not uncommon for clients who have problems with their hearing aids to drop by without an appointment and expect to be squeezed into the schedule for a brief visit.

6. **The clinical site.** The university clinic often has more flexibility in scheduling clients than other sites such as hospitals or private practices. The university clinic is more likely to gear appointments to meet the needs of the students, whereas the private practice gears appointments to the needs and demands of clients.

University Clinic Schedules

All clinical settings are restricted by their hours of operation and influenced by the availability and scheduling needs of their clients. Scheduling at the university clinic also is heavily influenced by the availability of clinical supervisors and student clinicians.

University clinics with large audiology programs often offer audiological services on a daily basis, Monday through Friday. Smaller university clinics may have more restricted schedules and may offer audiological services on only 1 or 2 days per week. They might still provide quality, comprehensive services. As a rule, university clinics operate during the regular business hours of the university. Therefore, clinical appointments might be scheduled any time between 8:00 A.M. to 5:00 P.M., Monday through Friday. Diagnostic appointments may be scheduled from 1 to 2 hours, depending on clients' needs and the student clinician's level of experience. Additional appointments, such as appointments for hearing aids, electronystagmography, auditory brainstem response testing, or follow-up appointments also will vary depending on the complexity of the client's problems, tasks to be completed, and the skill level of the student clinician.

You may be given your clinical assignment the semester before beginning your clinical practicum. As a general rule, you will attend a clinical meeting at the beginning of the term and receive your clinical assignment. Initially, you may be assigned clients for a few hours each week. The amount of time may be expanded as the term progresses, as you gain clinical experience, and as more clients contact the clinic. Occasionally, if there is a lull in clients seeking services, you may have some days without appointments. You can use these rare opportunities to sharpen your clinical expertise by practicing with different equipment, reviewing charts, and testing other student clinicians.

Beginning student clinicians generally are assigned one clinical supervisor. Occasionally, you will have more than one. At the beginning of the semester, your supervisors will discuss clinical policies and procedures, inform you of their expectations, tell you the schedule for clinic meetings, and answer questions you may have regarding your clinical assignment. After you meet with your clinical supervisor, you will begin seeing clients.

The clinic secretary schedules clients based on a prearranged plan with the clinic supervisor and clinic director. The clinic secretary will write the name of each client scheduled in an appointment book. You should check the appointment book regularly to ensure you are prepared for each appointment. Depending on the number of days and hours you are involved in clinical practicum, you may need to check the appointment book once a week or several times a day.

Hospital Schedules

A hospital clinic's schedule will coincide with regular business hours of the hospital. Again, appointments will be made Monday through Friday, between 8:00 A.M. and 5:00 P.M. If you are completing a full-time internship in a hospital setting, you may see clients any time during these hours. You will, of course, have a break for lunch and some time assigned for completing reports and other professional duties.

If you work with inpatients, your schedule may change depending on the needs and other services your patients receive. For example, you may be scheduled to perform a bedside audiological screening of a patient who was admitted with a traumatic brain injury; however, when you arrive in the patient's room he or she may be receiving nursing services. You may need to wait a few minutes or return at a later time.

Your hospital schedule also may include attendance at "rounds" or "grand rounds," during which the medical team discusses evaluation plans, results, and treatment plans for assigned patients. Rounds may take place in patients' rooms or in a conference room. A physician is the leader and facilitator during rounds and asks team members for impressions, comments, and treatment recommendations.

Clinical schedules in the outpatient setting will be similar to those in other clinics. Clients will be scheduled by the clinic secretary or receptionist, and you will be given a schedule of your appointments, usually on a daily basis. Appointments are usually 30 minutes to 1 hour in duration. During this time, you must complete your audiological assessment, discuss the results and recommendations with the client, complete any necessary charting, and complete any required billing forms. You also may be required to fit hearing aids during this time, if recommended. As part of your weekly schedule, time is allowed for report writing, staff meetings, and contact with other professionals.

In some hospitals, audiologists divide their time between in- and outpatients. Being flexible and using good time management skills will help you have a successful internship.

School Schedules

Educational audiologists employed by the public schools often have a variety of duties. These duties include performing hearing evaluations and immittance testing, recommending and servicing auditory trainers, and providing inservices to parents, teachers, school nurses, and school administrators. Although some educational audiologists are based at a single school, most are itinerant serving several schools. The itinerant educational audiologist often spends much of the day traveling from one school to the next, especially when schools are many miles apart.

To receive the services of the educational audiologist, students must be identified as deaf or hard-of-hearing and eligible for services. Individual Educational Plans (IEPs) are developed for these children including the services of an educational audiologist. The audiologist then develops his or her own schedule for providing services. The audiologist, of course, is aware of other scheduled activities of the children and arranges for their schedules to be disrupted as little as possible.

Regardless of the internship settings included in your daily schedule, you may need to coordinate your scheduling with other professionals providing service to your clients. Therefore, you often have to coordinate your schedule with those of other professionals. For instance, you may need to arrange a meeting with the school speech-language pathologist or the educator of the deaf to discuss the management plan for a child you have assessed.

Staffing Clients

Staffing clients is necessary whether it is done formally or informally. Formal staffing involves a specific time set aside for discussing clients, their evaluation results, and their management programs. Formal staffings may be scheduled each day of clinic, once a week, or even monthly. Informal staffing occurs whenever two or more professionals involved in delivering services to a client speak to one another about the client. Informal staffing may be face-to-face. For example, the educational audiologist and the school nurse may discuss a child's needs when the child is brought to the nurse's office to be seen by the itinerant audiologist. Much informal staffing occurs via the telephone. For example, the audiologist may telephone the client's physician to report the results of the hearing test and to discuss management options.

Formal staffing serves a variety of purposes. The time may be used to discuss client needs, plan evaluations, and discuss management options. In the university practicum situation, cases from the previous session often are reviewed and cases to be seen in the next session planned. Another purpose of staffing may be to involve other professionals in the management of the client. For example, a preschool-aged child with a hearing impairment may need the services of a speech-language pathologist and day-care placement for socialization. The day-care teacher, parents, speech-language pathologist, and audiologist may meet to discuss and to anticipate the child's needs. Yet another purpose of staffing is to educate staff concerning unusual or rare case studies. Staff meetings also may serve other purposes, for example, to introduce clinicians to new procedures. Whatever the primary purpose of staffings, they are usually formally scheduled in most facilities.

ASHA has recognized the importance of staffing in clinical practice. ASHA allows you to count 25 clinical clock hours of staffing "in which evaluation, treatment and/or recommendations are discussed or formulated, with or without the client present" (*Asha,* 1990d, p. 112).

Assessment of Clients

Clients may be seen for assessment for several reasons. Some clients may be scheduled for audiological evaluations as part of a routine annual physical examinations. Other clients may have failed hearing screenings performed at their schools or workplaces. Others may have difficulty understanding other people's speech and seek services on their own. Some children may be referred by their classroom teachers because they have difficulty following directions during class. Your initial assessment of these and other clients will help determine if an audiological disorder exists, if additional testing is needed, or if intervention is indicated.

Audiologic assessment and assessment of communicative needs of persons with hearing impairment will be described in Part III. The following section provides an overview of common procedures in an evaluation session.

Assessments at the University Clinic

Initial evaluation typically consists of obtaining a case history, client interview, screening for speech and language problems, otoscopy, immittance testing, pure-tone and speech testing. Procedures and tests will vary depending on the client and his or her complaints. A few steps are common to all assessments.

1. **Obtain a case history.** At the university clinic, you may receive the case history from the client prior to seeing the client. In some settings, you and the client will complete the case history together during the initial interview. Regardless of when and how you obtain the case history, it is an important part of the evaluation process. The case history suggests directions for testing, indicates the extent of the client's concern about the problem, and gives relevant medical, educational, and social information. Specifically, case histories include client identification data (e.g., name, address, telephone number, age, and insurance carrier); medical information, including a history of health and illnesses and current and past medications of interest, and other health professionals the client has seen or is seeing; the client's education; and, in the case of children, prenatal, birth, and developmental information, current school status and classroom performance; social information, including a history of the family structure; individuals available to assist the client; types of activities the client is and was involved in; the social and personal effects of the hearing impairment; and so forth.

2. **Interview the client.** As previously mentioned, you may obtain the case history during the client interview. During the interview, you will clarify any questions you have about the client's history and respond to any questions or concerns expressed by the client. Many variables influence the length of the interview. For example, if the client has a complex medical history, you will need to ask more and detailed questions. If the client is a young child whose teacher has complained that the child does not seem to listen in class, you will need to spend time gaining information about the child's academic performance, social interactions in and out of school, family interactions, and an in-depth medical and developmental history.

The most successful interviews allow the client to feel comfortable in both sharing information and asking questions. Clients may not always tell you information that you would consider diagnostically significant, because they do not think it is relevant to their problem. If you first establish rapport with your clients, they will feel more at ease and be more open in responding to your inquiries. To help your clients feel comfortable, they should be told what to expect during the evaluation. When you first meet your clients, introduce yourself and identify your role in the clinic. Briefly, give an overview of what you will be doing. For example, "First, I'm going to ask you a few questions, then I'll begin the hearing tests. After I have completed the tests, I'll discuss the results with you." Also, asking open-ended questions often results in clients giving you more information. Instead of asking, "Do you have trouble hearing in noisy environments?" you might say, "Tell me what types of hearing problems you have in noisy places, like parties, or noisy restaurants."

Write down or tape record all information relevant to the client's hearing. You may think you can remember all the client has said, but later you may forget important statements the client or the family members made to you. If tape recording, obtain the client's permission.

3. **Screen the client's speech and language.** ASHA's PSB guidelines require that speech and language screenings be routinely performed as part of the audiological assessment. Experienced clinicians often complete this screening informally during the client interview. Information about the client's articulation, fluency, voice, and language can be obtained from the client's conversational speech. Less experienced clinicians and student clinicians may follow a formal protocol. Regardless of the format you use to identify speech and language problems, be sure to refer your client to a speech-language pathologist if your screening indicates a need for a complete speech and language evaluation.

4. **Administer otoscopy.** Visual inspection of the ear is the first direct observation made in the audiologic test battery. Appropriate diagnosis depends on accurate evaluation, accurate evaluation results from careful observation. Otoscopy is more than a cursory examination of the ear canal and identifying the cone of light.

Before approaching the ear canal, observe the auricle and identify the major landmarks. Are all present? Are there fistulae? **Fistulae** are abnormal ducts or canals. Is the ear canal round? Can the canal be collapsed by pressing in front of the tragus? Does the texture of the skin appear normal? Are there suspicious growths? Does the canal appear abnormally narrow? After answering these questions and noting any unusual features, insert the speculum of the otoscope slowly into the ear. While inserting the speculum, observe the texture and color of the canal wall. Are there abrasions, sores, or abnormal growths? Is there excessive **cerumen** (ear wax) that obstructs your view? If so, does it need to be removed before continuing? Which direction does the ear canal travel? Are the bends in the canal marked or slight? Is the canal excessively hairy?

After carefully examining the canal, observe the tympanic membrane. Is the handle of the malleus visible? Is the cone of light in the anterior inferior quadrant? Is the membrane pearly gray? Is the membrane red or does it have a bluish cast? Are there holes in the membrane? Does the membrane appear scarred? After answering these questions, examine the other ear in a similar manner. Both ears should be relatively the same in appearance. If they are not, note the differences for future reference. Once the otoscopic examination is completed, you may proceed to immittance testing. As otoacoustic emission testing becomes standard clinical procedure, many audiologist will choose to do it next, especially with children. However, otoacoustic emission testing is not yet available in many settings and immittance testing will continue to provide useful diagnostic information.

5. **Immittance testing.** This test requires insertion of a probe tip into the ear. The tip must fit tightly to create an airtight seal. Otoscopy must precede the insertion of anything into the ear canal. In immittance testing, **dynamic compliance functions** (tympanometry), **static compliance,** and **acoustic reflex data** are obtained. Interpretation of the immittance battery is the subject of academic course work and is covered in several texts, so that information will not be repeated here.

In the beginning, students seem to err to the extremes in probe tip insertion. Many are overly concerned with causing the client discomfort and choose too small a tip. They then proceed to lose the tip in the ear canal or fail to obtain a seal. Other students select tips that are too large and attempt to cram them into the ear canal despite the client's protests. Do not despair. It will not be long before you gain experience in selecting and inserting the appropriate probe tip under supervision.

6. **Administer pure-tone testing.** You will want to have mastered pure-tone air- and bone-conduction test procedures and be able to mask when necessary. Some off-campus practicum settings do not routinely administer bone-conduction tests. However, most university clinics require bone-conduction testing. The experienced clinician may think bone-conduction tests unnecessary in light of immittance results. You need to administer many bone conduction tests before you have the experience to interpret hearing loss type correctly without them.

Pure-tone air-conduction averages are computed for 500, 1000, and 2000 Hertz (Hz). These averages are later compared to speech reception measures to estimate test validity.

7. **Administer speech tests.** Speech tests in the initial battery are of two types: speech reception tests and word recognition tests. Speech reception tests are threshold measures, and word recognition tests are measures of speech understanding.

Speech reception tests may measure Speech Threshold (ST) by finding the lowest level at which the client can repeat back bisyllabic words. In lieu of an ST, a speech detection threshold (SDT) may be obtained by finding the lowest level at which the client signals that bisyllabic words are heard. The SDT is about 8 dB more sensitive than the ST. When the ST and the pure-tone average are compared, a measure of test validity is obtained. Pure-tone air-conduction tests are considered valid when they agree with ST results within 8 dB.

Word recognition measures have been variously referred to as speech discrimination scores (SDS), word discrimination scores (WDS), and other names. "Word recognition tests" probably is a better descriptive term for the materials used and the responses required of the client. You should administer materials at suprathreshold levels. The level chosen depends on the information needed. For example, if you want to know how well the client understands speech at normal conversational levels, present the words at 50 dB HL. If you want to know the client's maximum percent correct score, present the words at the phonetically balanced maximum (PB Max) for that list. Performance-intensity (PI) functions are most helpful in assessing a client's word recognition abilities at different presentation levels.

Initial audiologic assessment in the university clinic generally includes the case history, an interview, screening for speech and language problems, otoscopy, immittance, pure-tone, and speech testing. Complete batteries of tests and standard procedures are emphasized. You must practice complete batteries and standard procedures before you become comfortable with the interrelationships between the tests and know how to interpret them. Once you become comfortable with the complete, standard battery, you can abbreviate the battery and use other procedures without sacrificing diagnostic validity.

Reassessment of Clients

Clients may be reassessed on an annual basis. Before you begin the actual testing, you should update the client's case history to determine relevant changes in the clients medical, educational, or social status. The client's previous test results and the updated case history will influence the extent of your current testing.

Establishing a Working Relationship with the Client and the Family

As a student audiologist, you may see a client only once, or you may have clients that you see weekly for several weeks. To maximize your effectiveness as a clinician and enhance your intervention, you must quickly establish an effective working relationship with the client and, if appropriate, the client's family. You will want your clients to share clinically relevant information readily with you, comply with your recommendations regarding needed services, and follow through on directions, such as care of hearing aids. Do not assume that, because someone has sought audiology services, he or she is prepared to admit he or she has a hearing problem. Also, there will be clients who want you to perform miracles. In most instances, it takes patience, understanding, and perseverance to provide appropriate service. For example, it is very difficult for parents who have just been told that their child has a significant hearing loss to understand all the ramifications of the child's hearing loss immediately. The parents may be angry, hurt, or disbelieving. Individuals are more likely to discuss information with you and comply with directions when they trust and respect your skills, and understand the reasons you ask certain questions or give certain directions. The following section will help you establish working relationships with your clients.

1. **Be prepared for each session.** Nothing turns a client off faster than a clinician who appears unprepared. Although the client knows you are a student clinician, he or she still expects to receive quality care. In fact, because you are a student clinician, you may have to appear more professional and better prepared than the professional who can rely on his or her credentials. You do not have a professional reputation yet and will have only about an hour to establish your reputation with the client. Check your equipment in advance to make sure everything is working properly. Know where all the supplies you will need are kept. Have handy extra supplies that you may need. Review your testing procedures, any information related to your client's disorder, and intervention techniques before you see the client.

2. **Introduce yourself.** Tell the client that you will be providing the services under the supervision of an audiologist. If your supervisor is present, introduce your supervisor to the client. Never misrepresent your professional training. If you are well prepared and appear assured, the client will have confidence in you and understand if you need to say, "I'm not sure about that, let me check with my supervisor." Also,

be sure to ask your supervisor when you have questions. Do not try to bluff your way through the session.

3. **Tell the client what to expect from the session.** Describe the sequence of the session. As you begin each new activity or test, tell the client, or the parent, what test you are giving and what types of information the test will give you. You do not need to give a detailed description of each activity, just an overview using common terms.

4. **Avoid the use of jargon.** Speak in simple language, but do not patronize clients. In other words, adjust your vocabulary and explanations to the level your client can understand. If you are working with a physician, use medical terminology in your discussion without explaining what each term refers to. If you are working with a client who has had little education, describe your activities or disorders using professional terminology, but explain each term in everyday language. When you are working with children, use simple descriptions and analogies that children are likely to understand.

5. **Early in the session, ask if the client has any questions.** Tell the client to feel free to ask questions throughout the session. If you are unsure how to reply to a client's question, ask your supervisor.

6. **Follow-up with a phone call.** Take a few minutes out of each day to follow-up with phone calls to clients you think may have questions or problems.

Report Writing

Report writing is an important aspect of the profession. Although you should learn to write reports quickly and concisely, you should learn to write them well. Written reports reflect your professional skills. People who have never met you will judge your clinical abilities on how and what you say in your reports. You may write different types of reports. After a diagnostic session, you will write an assessment or diagnostic report which gives a comprehensive description of the results of the evaluation session and your recommendations. A reassessment report may be written when a client is seen a second time. This report provides current test information and, generally, compares this information with previous test results. Treatment plans which may be written for clients receiving management services include an overview of the disorder and goals of treatment. If you are employed in the public schools, you may be required to write Individualized Education Programs (IEPs). IEPs are required for all children ages 3 through 21 years of age who are enrolled in special education. You also may be required to write information for an Individual Family Service Plan (IFSP), which is written for children birth through 2 years of age.

Each practicum site will have its own writing format and procedures. However, some writing guidelines can be used across settings. These are discussed in the following section.

General Guidelines for Report Writing

Report writing is an important skill for students to master. Your clinical report not only reflects your knowledge and professional skill, but serves as a written documentation of services provided. Your reports must be clear and concise, yet provide sufficient information to be useful to the reader. Much of your work as an audiologist will be in collaboration with other professionals, and you must learn to communicate effectively with them. For example, you will routinely receive referrals from and refer clients to ear, nose, and throat specialists (otorhinolaryngologists). You also may frequently communicate with a client's pediatrician or family physician. The school speech-language pathologist who is working with one of your clients who has a hearing impairment will want current information on the status of the client's hearing. Although some of your communication with allied service providers will be verbal, you often will send a written report as a more efficient means of communication. Because documentation and accountability are heavily emphasized for health care providers, well written reports provide excellent documentation.

There are many aspects to good report writing. Of course, one of the first aspects is having accurate data to write about. After you have obtained the information you want to document, you must organize and report it in a clear and concise manner. To maximize the effectiveness of the information you report, grammar, spelling, and punctuation must be accurate; and the report should be neatly prepared. Initially, student clinicians spend much time writing reports. Do not let messy reports decrease the impact your report has on the reader. The content and format of your reports will be discussed at each of your practicum sites. However, some general rules you can follow in writing reports include:

1. Organize and present information in a logical sequence.
2. Use complete sentences.
3. Spell words correctly. Check the spelling of words you are unfamiliar with or unsure of before including them in your report.
4. Punctuate all sentences correctly.
5. State information clearly. Do not write contradictory or nebulous statements.
6. Detail important information. Present essential information concisely, but with sufficient detail.
7. Do not make inferential jumps. Make sure that your clinical impressions are substantiated by quantifiable data.
8. Use nonsexist and culturally nonbiased language.
9. Avoid the use of jargon. If you must use some jargon, determine whether it is necessary to include a brief description of what it means in the report.
10. Do not use qualifiers such as *like, very, rather,* and so on.
11. Follow the reporting format described by your supervisor.
12. Use the required type of paper. If a specific paper is not required, avoid the use of erasable paper or colored paper that is difficult to photocopy.
13. Use a good ribbon when typing or printing your report. Print should be dark enough for reports to easily be read and photocopied.
14. Proofread your reports before submitting them. Do not let careless mistakes slip by you. To catch typographical errors, sometimes you need to allow time between when you first write your report and when your proof it.

As previously mentioned, different clinical sites will have different report writing requirements. The length, number, format, and style of reports required will vary depending on your practicum site. Your clinical supervisor will provide you with report writing guidelines for your clinical site. The following section gives some suggestions and guidelines for writing reports.

Audiological Report

After you have completed your audiological evaluation, you will write an evaluation or assessment report. The evaluation report summarizes pertinent client history, assessment procedures and results, clinical impressions, and recommendations. The report also documents the client's audiological status prior to intervention and serves as a written record to which future data can be compared. The evaluation report also may be used as a method of communication with other professionals or agencies. For example, clients may ask you to send copies of their reports to their physicians. Insurance companies may require that a copy of the diagnostic report be submitted with your billing. Although the reporting format will vary depending on your practicum site, the following information generally should be included in each evaluation report.

1. **Client identification data.** Include in each report the client's name, age, date of birth, and the date of the evaluation. Probably, you also will want to include the client's telephone number and address.

2. **Background information.** Give a brief summary of the client's history and his or her reason for seeking your services. If applicable, include the name of the person who referred the client to you in this section. If your client received previous audiological services at another agency, include a statement about those services.

3. **Test results.** Describe the assessment procedures used and the results obtained. For example, "standard pure-tone, immittance, and speech tests were administered" is a description of assessment procedures. "The results of these tests indicate normal hearing" is a statement about results obtained.

4. **Clinical impressions or observations.** Observations that are relevant to test findings are stated in this section. For example, "the client reported that he was knocked unconscious in an explosion at work" is a relevant observation.

5. **Recommendations.** Make your recommendations. Your recommendations must be based on data that have been detailed in the section on assessment results and clinical impressions. Do not make recommendations that your data do not justify.

6. **Signature and date of report.** The person responsible for the information in the report should sign and date the report. Student clinicians will sign their reports, and their supervisors also will sign the reports.

Record Keeping Procedures

You will be responsible for maintaining a variety of records throughout your academic and professional career. As a student clinician, you will be required to maintain both your client records and your log of clinical practicum hours earned accurately and legibly. The following sections give an overview of some of your record keeping responsibilities. Your clinical supervisor will give you more specific information.

Client Files

To provide high quality and efficient clinical services, client records must be complete, accurate, neat, and orderly. Files must be maintained in a manner that allows important information to be retrieved easily. Although the office staff initially will be responsible for putting your client's file together, you will be responsible for the content and maintenance of the file. You will have the most contact with the client while performing the necessary tests, making clinical recommendations, and providing consultation and follow-up services. You will routinely write and update information in the client's file. Remember that all reports and records (such as audiograms) must be signed by both the student clinician and the clinical supervisor.

At all times, you should protect the confidentiality of information maintained in client files. Therefore, client files must be maintained in a locking file cabinet. Client files should not be removed from the clinic area. For example, do not take client files with you to the cafeteria, and never take client files home. Do not leave client files on counters or unattended in the clinic area. If you cannot locate a client's file, notify the clinic secretary immediately.

Follow your clinical practicum site's guidelines for recording clinical activities, filing reports, and updating client information. If you have any questions about these procedures, ask your clinical supervisor. According to ASHA's Professional Service Board (1984), client records should include the following information:

1. **Information for client identification.** Each client's file should contain the client's telephone number, address, file number, insurance carrier, place of employment of the client or client's parent, and so forth.

2. **The individual or agency that referred the client for services.** It is important to have the name of the referral source because clients often want copies of their reports sent to the referral source. It is also a good business practice to acknowledge the referral by sending a letter to the person who referred the client to you. You

also may need referral information for data collection, or if you have any questions about your client that the referral source may be able to answer.

3. **Information related to your clinical services from other agencies.** For example, this may include copies of medical reports, educational evaluations, speech and language evaluations, or audiological evaluations completed at other facilities.

4. **The name of the audiologist responsible for providing service.** In the case of student clinicians, the names of both the student clinician and the clinical supervisor should be noted in the file.

5. **All reports.** Originals of all diagnostic reports and management plans should be included.

6. **A method of tracking clinical services.** This often is a chronological log that tracks all clinical services, including referrals, that the client received while at your facility.

7. **A signed and dated authorization for release of information.** All adult clients and parents or guardians of child clients should sign a release form.

Practicum Hours

As you know, you are required to earn a minimum number of clinical practicum clock hours for graduation and for ASHA certification. Some universities require additional clock hours beyond ASHA's minimum standards. Regardless of the clinical clock hour requirements at your university, these hours must be documented. Each university will have procedures and forms for students to use in recording and reporting clinical clock hours. You should follow these procedures. You are responsible for documenting your clinical practicum hours. If you are unsure which activities can be counted as clinical hours, refer to Chapter 1 or ask your clinical supervisor. The more detailed your record of practicum hours, the easier it will be for you to complete the paperwork required for ASHA certification and state licensure.

Working with Other Professionals

Both student and professional audiologists work with other professionals. Your clinical setting will influence the amount of interaction you have with other professionals and the kinds of professionals you generally work with. For example, if your practicum site is a local elementary school, you may work closely with teachers, school-based speech-language pathologists, and school nurses. However, if your site is a Veteran's Administration hospital, you will have little interaction with teachers, but work closely with otorhinolaryngologists and other medical and surgical specialists. Regardless of your practicum site, to provide the best service possible, you should learn to work with other professionals. To develop an effective working relationship with other professionals, you must know what their roles are in relation to the services you provide. The following is an overview of the roles of some of the professions you may work with.

Health Professionals

1. **Primary care physician.** Primary care physicians are the gatekeepers for health maintenance organizations, professional provider groups, and other forms of prepaid health care. These physicians frequently are the first professionals consulted about hearing loss. Primary care physicians most often are family practitioners and internists for adults and pediatricians for children. These physicians do not routinely screen for hearing problems, and the medical environment is not conducive to identifying hearing problems the patient is not aware of or concerned about. On the other hand, primary care physicians consistently refer patients who present with complaints of hearing or speech problems. Physicians may refer these patients to ear, nose, and throat specialists, audiologists, or hearing aid dispensers. A referral from the primary care physician most often is required for health insurance groups to pay for hearing services.

The primary care physician often will refer a patient with a complaint of hearing loss to the ear specialist. As primary care physicians develop professional relationships with independent audiologists in private practice, referrals directly to audiologists may increase.

2. **Otorhinolaryngologist.** Frequently referred to as ear, nose, and throat specialists (ENTs), otorhinolaryngologists are physicians with specialized training in disorders of the ear, nose, and throat. Audiologists often works closely with these specialists.

3. **Family practitioners.** General practitioners who treat all members of a family.

4. **Pediatrician.** A physician who has specialized training in childhood disorders and treatment.

5. **Neurologist.** A physician who is a specialist in diseases of the nervous system.

6. **Orthodontist.** A dentist with specialized training in dental abnormalities.

7. **Oral and maxillofacial surgeon.** A specialist who deals with oral and facial structures and their surgical repair.

8. **Physical therapist (PT).** The registered physical therapist (RPT) evaluates and provides intervention for disorders related to physical and musculoskeletal injuries.

9. **Occupational therapist (OT or OTR).** Occupational therapists are primarily employed in hospitals or skilled nursing facilities. The occupational therapist evaluates individuals' daily living skills and provides intervention if indicated. Daily living skills involve activities such as eating, dressing, cooking, and bathing. Certain occupational therapists specialize. For example, an occupational therapist might specialize in the rehabilitation of hands. It is not unusual for OTs to be involved in training clients in the use of adaptive living devices to help clients live more independently. These devices may include modified cooking equipment (such as stoves with special controls) or adaptive equipment for independent dressing.

10. **Clinical and educational psychologists.** Clinical psychologists work with personal, behavioral, and emotional problems. Educational psychologists work with school children who have learning and academic problems.

11. **Speech-language pathologist.** The speech-language pathologist is a specialist in the identification and treatment of speech, language, and voice disorders. Many speech-language pathologists also assess and treat disorders of swallowing and feeding. The audiologist and speech-language pathologist interact frequently.

12. **Registered nurse (RN).** The registered nurse works closely with patients and, in the hospital setting, is the professional who provides most of the medical care prescribed by the physician.

13. **Social worker.** The social worker is a professional with training in human behavior and counseling. The social worker often acts as a liaison between families and public service organizations and as a patient advocate. In the medical setting, the social worker is a member of the hospital's rehabilitation team.

14. **Vocational rehabilitation counselor.** A specialist who counsels people with employment-related problems and finds employment-related resources for people with special needs.

15. **Hearing aid dispenser.** In years past, before otolaryngologists began dispensing hearing aids, ear specialists and some primary

care physicians referred patients with hearing losses directly to hearing aid dispensers. A hearing aid dispenser is a person licensed to sell hearing aids. There is an increasing trend for physicians to refer to hearing aid dispensers who also happen to be licensed audiologists.

Educational Specialists

1. **Adaptive physical education specialist.** These specialists work with individuals who have motor disabilities. They have specialized training in physical education and develop and implement physical education programs for individuals with disabilities.

2. **Educational audiologist.** An audiologist who works in public schools and specializes in the assessment and management of hearing impairment as it relates to children's education.

3. **Principal.** The administrator of the school. As an educational audiologist, you may not work closely with the principal. However, the principal will influence your service delivery in the school setting.

4. **School nurse.** A school nurse is responsible for maintaining students' health records and providing first-aid to children. At many schools, the school nurse also provides vision and hearing screenings.

5. **Special education teacher.** There are many types of special education teachers including the teachers of the Hearing Impaired (HI), teachers of the Severely Emotionally Disturbed (SED), and teachers of the Learning Handicapped (LH). Educational audiologists work closely with teachers of the hearing impaired.

6. **Speech-language pathologist.** The speech-language pathologist employed in the public schools evaluates and treats children who have communication disorders. The educational audiologist is likely to work closely with the school speech-language pathologist.

As you can see, there are many professionals you may work with. To maximize your effectiveness as an audiologist, you need to establish good working relationships with other professionals. An essential ingredient in developing a good working relationship with other professionals is mutual respect. Make sure that you provide good services and refer your clients only to other professionals who provide equally good services. It is also important to communicate regularly and promptly with other professionals. If an otologist telephones you regarding a client, return the call promptly. To avoid conflicts with other professionals and to uphold the ASHA Code of Ethics, provide only services you are qualified to provide.

In the following parts of this book, you will learn about specific components of service delivery in audiology. Part II deals with hearing conservation, Part III with diagnosis, and Part IV with management of auditory problems.

Part II

Hearing Conservation

I n Part I, you learned the basic structure of clinical practicum in audiology and some of the rules and guidelines you must follow. The initial audiologic practicum experiences offered for speech-language pathologists and audiologists vary among training programs. In some programs, students in speech and language pathology are involved primarily with identification audiometry and school hearing conservation programs. Students in audiology also gain experience with identification audiometry and hearing conservation. However, audiology students may extend their experiences to hearing conservation programs in the community outside of schools, to health fairs, senior citizen facilities, hospital-based neonatal hearing screening programs, and industry.

In Part II, you will be introduced to strategies for conducting hearing conservation programs. A strategy can be defined as a careful plan or method by which to achieve a goal. Therefore, in Part II, you will be provided with methods to accomplish your goal of successfully completing audiology practicum in hearing conservation.

6

An Overview of Hearing Conservation

H earing conservation programs are an integral activity
in most audiologic practices and have three common goals:

- identifying existing hearing loss
- preventing hearing loss
- educating the population to care for their hearing.

Identification audiometry in the hearing conservation setting
may involve hearing screening or testing. Its primary purpose is the
identification of people at risk for hearing loss. Students in audiologic
practicum may be called on to screen or test the hearing of a variety
of school-age children, the general public, including senior citizens and
neonates, or workers exposed to excessive noise.

Sometimes, identification audiometry occurs in the primary practicum setting. At other times, students may be required to travel to
off-campus facilities.

Students in audiology practicum are required to participate in
activities designed to prevent hearing loss. Recommendations for noise
reduction through sound treatment is one activity designed to prevent

hearing loss from excess exposure to noise. Another activity in which practicum students may participate is fitting hearing protection.

Besides participating in identification audiometry and the prevention of hearing loss, the student in practicum may be asked to educate people on how to care for their hearing. For example, the student may be asked to make a presentation to workers concerning the effects of noise on hearing or to offer an in-service to school or nursing home personnel. **In-services** in the area of hearing conservation are educational training programs designed to describe normal hearing, explain hearing loss, and identify hearing conservation goals for a specific facility.

The student may be asked to conduct the entire hearing conservation program, including making the initial contacts, administering the program, and completing follow-up activities. When given the responsibility for executing a total hearing conservation program, the student has an opportunity to learn important administrative and public relations skills. Most importantly, conducting an effective hearing conservation program requires planning.

Planning a Hearing Conservation Program

Relationships between facilities in need of conservation programs and those that provide them originate in a variety of ways. The facility may have identified a need and contacted the audiology service program with a request for services. Often a university audiology program has contacted a facility offering to provide a hearing conservation program. By so doing, the university clinic can provide students in practicum with experience conducting hearing conservation programs and clinical contact with persons in specific age groups. The contracting facility may benefit from receiving a high-quality service at substantially lower cost by contracting that service from a university. When a facility has expressed interest in a hearing conservation program, an appointment is made to meet with the facility administrator and tour its facilities. A hearing conservation program is then developed for the facility.

Several problems arise when developing hearing conservation programs. Many of the common problems that you will encounter are enumerated below. Following the problems are solutions. In some instances, specific procedures are outlined to implement the suggested solutions. Solutions other than those suggested may be appropriate. You and your supervisor may prefer another solution to a problem or implement the solutions suggested. The purpose of presenting issues related to hearing conservation in this format is to provide the beginning student with as much specific information about what to do in various situations as is possible.

Problem 6-1. The objectives of the hearing conservation program are not clear.

Solution 6-1. Identify the program objectives before implementing the hearing conservation program and include them in the introductory section of the report on the program to the facility for which it is conducted.

The objective of an effective hearing conservation program is to pass individuals with hearing at or better than the screening level. The program identifies individuals with hearing worse than the screening level for follow-up. A program that does not identify those with hearing loss cannot be effective. A program that identifies those with normal hearing as having hearing loss over-refers and cannot be considered effective.

Many facilities do not place a high priority on hearing conservation programs. Hearing conservation programs in schools draw students away from classes and interrupt scheduled learning activities. Likewise, programs in the community disrupt people's daily schedules. Hearing conservation programs in industry may take a worker away from the production line. Therefore, to be effective, participants in a hearing conservation setting should be able to get in and out of a facility with as little disruption to regularly scheduled activities as possible.

Problem 6-2. A facility you have contacted wants to know the benefits of conducting a hearing conservation program.

Solution 6-2. Offer reasons why a hearing conservation program may be beneficial.

Society is at risk if hearing loss goes undetected in the population. One reason for offering a hearing conservation program is that hearing loss represents a liability for society. School-age children with hearing impairments have difficulty achieving their potentials and represent an avoidable cost to society as a whole. Although the human cost resulting from hearing loss is difficult to measure, some costs can be measured in lost income and taxes not paid by a low-wage earning adult. Other costs can be measured in terms of money spent on social programs for adults who are unable to support themselves.

Another reason to offer hearing conservation programs is that some population subgroups may be at greater risk for hearing loss than the community at large. Workers exposed to high noise levels are at significant risk for hearing loss. Military personnel have a greater risk for hearing loss than civilians. Everyone has a right to a safe and healthy working environment. Society has an obligation to conserve the hearing and the quality of life of these individuals. The benefits of the hearing conservation program should be stated in the introductory section of the report on the program given to the facility when the program is completed.

Problem 6-3. Facility expectations of services are not known.

Solution 6-3. Clarify facility expectations.

Administrators and staff perceive the purpose of hearing screening as identification of hearing problems and expect that hearing problems identified by the screening will be treated. Practicum assignments are usually for a semester or quarter at a time. It is important to allow enough time during the practicum assignment for proper follow-up because the reasonable expectations of the administration and staff of the facility should be met.

Problem 6-4. Cooperation from facility personnel must be ensured.

Solution 6-4. Conduct in-service information sessions for the facility staff and the program's target population.

The person in charge of the hearing conservation program is usually responsible for educating facility personnel regarding conservation of hearing and identification audiometry. The educational component of the program involves educating the facility's administration and staff to increase their understanding of and support for the hearing conservation program. Education also involves teaching the targeted population to recognize dangers to and how to care for their hearing. Students in practicum may not count hours of inservice presentations to staff as diagnostic clinical contact hours. However, they can count time spent educating the target population about hearing loss and conservation.

Education of the administrative personnel is accomplished in an initial meeting. Education of staff is accomplished best during a scheduled staff meeting. Staff meetings on the hearing conservation program should be held at the facility during regular hours. Allow up to one-half hour for the presentation, depending on the setting, and a few minutes to field questions. The presentation should encourage interaction. Staff personnel are a great resource in preparing those under their supervision to be screened, and great care should be taken to enlist their active participation in the program. Inservices for staff should take place a few days to a week before identification audiometry takes place. This allows the staff sufficient time to prepare themselves and those under their supervision for identification audiometry.

To the extent possible, the regular routine of the facility receiving hearing conservation services should not be disrupted. Therefore, educational sessions for staff should be scheduled in regular on-site staff meeting areas. For industrial workers, education may be best accomplished after testing in the testing area. Off-campus educational activities are difficult to justify in almost any hearing conservation setting.

Problem 6-5. Appropriate equipment for testing is not available on site.

Solution 6-5. Use portable audiometers.

Sound-treated mobile facilities capable of screening and testing several individuals automatically are available. Where hearing screening programs are mandated, such equipment may be purchased or services that have the equipment may be contracted. Typically, screening programs are conducted in offices, school classrooms, and senior citizen settings.

The testing space should be large enough to accommodate the number of testing or screening stations desired. Stations include space for the examiner as well as the individual being screened or tested. Stations must be located far enough apart so that activities at one station do not interfere with activities at the other stations.

Ideally, any activities normally scheduled in or around the space designated for screening should be suspended until the screening is completed. Some appliances make so much noise that they must be disconnected to provide an environment quiet enough to allow screening of hearing. It is necessary to inform the people whose activities will be disrupted by the screening well in advance, and, if possible, to provide acceptable alternatives.

Few clinical facilities can afford to purchase audiometers limited to identification audiometry for hearing conservation programs. Therefore, versatile audiometers that serve a variety of functions often are purchased. The most common instrument used in identification audiometry is the portable, single-channel, pure-tone audiometer. This machine has an on-off control, a control to select either the right or left earphone, a switch to turn the tone on or off, and a tone presentation bar or switch. In addition, there is a single frequency selector and a single intensity selector. The frequencies are in octave and selected half-octave intervals between 125 Hz and 8000 Hz. The intensities vary in 5 dB steps between 0 and 110 dB HL. The machine may or may not have bone-conduction testing capability. The machine must have been calibrated within the past 12 months and certified as having met ANSI 1969 standards. Only properly calibrated equipment should be used.

The number of audiometers needed to conduct identification audiometry in a particular setting depends on the number of individuals receiving services, the number of supervisors available, and the space available. If the test environment will accommodate more than one tester, two audiometers per supervisor may be used. It is always good to have a spare audiometer on hand in case one of the machines being used malfunctions.

Some facilities utilize immittance equipment when screening preschool and early elementary school-age children. Immittance screening picks up middle ear conditions that may be missed in pure-tone screening. The most common equipment used for immittance testing is the automatic screening device. Devices that combine immittance and pure-tone screening in one instrument also are available.

Problem 6-6. The amount of time needed to execute the hearing conservation program is not clear.

Solution 6-6. Estimate the time for education, identification, and follow-up services.

It is important to recognize certain time constraints. Days on which special programs are scheduled should be avoided when scheduling identification audiometry. The first and last days of the week often are more hectic than the middle three days of the typical work week.

Certain times of day are better to conduct identification audiometry than others. The best time of day for testing is setting-specific. Practicum students involved in scheduling of identification audiometry should determine the specific time constraints for the setting in which they are working.

Thirty minutes prior to beginning screening is ample time for setup. Allowing 5 to 10 minutes of time between preparations to screen and the beginning of screening is a good idea. During that time, screeners can use the restroom, get a drink, and relax. Beginning in a relaxed manner is important when initiating a 2 to 3 hour screening block.

The time needed to complete identification audiometry depends on several factors. A major factor is whether the audiometry consists of screening or threshold testing. The time needed to screen hearing varies with the cooperativeness of the individual being screened, the amount of screening to be done, and the organization, skill, and confidence of the tester. In most situations, total screening time for both ears should be under 5 minutes.

When identification audiometry involves establishing thresholds, the total testing time should be under 15 minutes. Total screening and testing time includes seating, instructing, administering the procedure to both ears, recording the data, and dismissing the individual.

Problem 6-7. Transportation for personnel and equipment may not be available.

Solution 6-7. Let one of the practicum students take the responsibility for transportation of personnel and equipment.

Often, two or more students in practicum are involved in a single hearing conservation program. Unless the supervisor acts as the director of the program, one of the students may be designated as *in-charge.* That student, then, is responsible for scheduling transportation. With the help of others, this student will arrange for transportation.

Many facilities do not have properly calibrated audiometers. Therefore, the audiologic team must carry its own audiometers to the facility. A student clinician may take the responsibility for this as well.

Problem 6-8. Individuals who are to receive identification audiometry must be moved to and from the testing site in an orderly manner.

Solution 6-8. Study the physical setting of the facility and design an efficient method of moving people to and from the testing site.

There are several effective methods of coordinating the movement of persons to and from the area in which the identification audiometry is being conducted. The method chosen should cause minimum disruption to the administration and the front office and create an even flow of persons.

Those administering the identification audiometry should not be responsible for bringing or returning persons to the test area. If the facility cannot provide someone to direct traffic flow, an additional person is necessary. If the additional person is a student in practicum, he or she cannot receive practicum credit for facilitating movement of persons to and from the identification audiometry area. Students facilitating movement of those to be tested can receive practicum credit by rotating with the students who are conducting the identification procedures. This arrangement spreads the available practicum hours equally among the participants and provides a change of activity for the practicum students involved.

As a general rule of thumb, individuals should be waiting to take the place of those being screened. Those who have been screened should return to their regularly scheduled activities and not loiter in the screening area. As one group is leaving, the group waiting should be moving into place to be screened, while newly arriving individuals wait their turn.

Problem 6-9. Who should be tested?

Solution 6-9. Find out the regulations or practices established in the practicum setting.

In the school setting, who is to be screened depends on an established schedule. Children may be screened every other year or every third year. If screening is a one-time event, all individuals at risk in the target population should be screened.

In other settings, most of the individuals in the setting will receive identification audiometry. In senior citizen settings all residents may be screened. In industry, all workers exposed to noise levels of 85 dB, as measured on the A scale (dBA) of a sound level meter, or greater must be tested. The A scale incorporates the threshold of human hearing as a low fence above which noise is measured. As a rule of thumb, the hearing of individuals exposed to these noise levels should be tested annually.

Problem 6-10. Appropriate types of test data must be determined.

Solution 6-10. Identification audiometry should include the frequencies and intensity levels specified by law, contained in ASHA Position Statements, or dictated by the purpose of the screening.

Screenings usually are conducted at a specific intensity level and at specific frequencies. ASHA has position statements and guidelines regarding pure-tone screening (ASHA, 1985) and immittance screening (ASHA, 1990a). State or federal laws also mandate intensity levels and specific frequencies to be screened in schools and in industry. Two other factors that influence the choice of frequencies and intensity levels are the:

- criteria used for hearing impairment
- ambient noise levels in the test area.

Specific criteria for the hearing levels used for pass/fail criteria vary depending on the site of hearing conservation. Therefore, they will be addressed in specific sections on different sites. Ambient noise levels are dealt with in more detail in the section on Noise Surveys.

Problem 6-11. Who will do the identification audiometry?

Solution 6-11. Screening and audiometric testing may be conducted by first semester practicum students.

For the students in practicum, the payoff is clinical clock hours. The clinical contact hours obtained will result primarily from identification audiometry.

To screen and test hearing effectively, the student in practicum must have completed study on the audiometer and its operation. In addition, the student should be familiar with variables that affect the validity of the testing situation. The student also should understand the various components of an effective hearing conservation program and how identification audiometry fits into the program. For all settings except the workplace, most of this information is provided in introductory course work in audiology.

Supervisors expect students to conduct the hearing conservation program in a professional and efficient manner. You are expected to be familiar with the equipment and with identification audiometry procedures. You are expected to behave in a confident, self-starting, and self-directed manner. You should be aware of the needs of the persons with whom you are working. You are expected to be open to supervision and to incorporate suggested changes into your behavior in a timely fashion. Dress should be appropriately professional.

You should be well-organized, efficient, and appear so. To be ready for the first individual presenting for screening, the persons doing the screening must have equipment set up, a listening check performed, forms and pencils ready for recording, and furniture arranged to facilitate screening.

Problem 6-12. The procedures for collecting audiometric data, writing reports, and making recommendations are not clear.

Solution 6-12. Appoint a member of the hearing conservation team to be responsible for assembling, organizing, and reporting data.

Often a student is appointed to take this responsibility. The clinical supervisor holds the final responsibility for the reports. The quality of the work submitted by students reflects on supervisors and, ultimately, on the clinical program that employs them.

Supervisors will be demanding. It often takes less time and effort for supervisors to do the report themselves, but a well-planned practicum experience will involve the student in practicum to the greatest degree possible.

The specific information to be reported for a particular hearing conservation program is related to the data needed for that setting. For example, state law may mandate that certain frequencies be screened at a particular intensity level for all public school children. In this case, all tested children, classified into those identified with hearing at or better than the screening limit and those with hearing worse than the screening limit, must be reported. You are encouraged to ask yourself, "What information do I need to report to enable those who conduct the next program to understand precisely what was done?"

In some hearing conservation settings, the reporting of data can be a sensitive issue. Some industries prefer that their own physicians counsel workers about the results. Reports, or information from reports, are confidential data and must be so treated.

Without exception, the agency or business contracting hearing conservation services should receive a report. For ongoing services, quarterly or semiannual reports may be appropriate. For general community hearing conservation programs, a report to the community through the news media may be appropriate. The audiology practice that provides hearing conservation services should always keep copies of reports for all hearing conservation programs conducted.

Reports must be timely. When reports are delayed, the facility that contracted the service may not have the results of the program in time to complete reports to government agencies, insurance companies, and referral sources. The facility that contracted the service should have the report in hand within 2 weeks from completion of the program. Multiple reports required of ongoing programs should be submitted at the quarterly or semiannual dates specified by the facility contracting the service. The importance of timely reporting cannot be overstressed.

Once screening is completed, follow-up services take place. Different settings may mandate specific follow-up schedules. For example, workers exposed to over 85 dBA of noise must be tested annually. Public school students who do not pass the screening often must be retested within 2 weeks. You need to be aware of follow-up requirements specific to the setting in which you are participating.

Follow-up services for individuals should be timely. Some programs recommend that individuals identified as at risk be brought to the clinical facility for diagnostic testing. Other programs refer the individual to sources of service other than the hearing conservation service provider. Whatever follow-up is appropriate, it should take place soon after the individual at risk for hearing problems is identified.

The purpose of identifying hearing problems in individuals is to make them and others significant to them aware of the hearing-impaired individual's needs and to recommend treatment. To determine what treatment is appropriate and, therefore, to whom the individual should be referred, diagnostic audiologic testing is often needed. Individuals who fail the pure-tone screening should be referred for diagnostic audiology.

Clinical facilities that conduct free hearing screening programs often have a secondary purpose of generating referrals to their own facilities. If the screening is being provided by more than one clinic, or if the clinic providing the service does not intend to provide follow-up services, referral to other facilities for follow-up services is necessary. Follow-up testing for those referred by the program will be to audiologic and medical offices in the geographic service area. As a part of the recommendations section in the report, some programs include a list of local service providers, their addresses, and telephone numbers.

The authors recommend that the person in charge of the hearing conservation program be directly responsible for referral and follow-up. Be aware that the facility being served must consent to follow-up services before they are initiated. The facility being served may insist on taking the entire responsibility for follow-up.

Problem 6-13. A person is exposed to potentially harmful levels of sound.

Solution 6-13. Provide hearing protection.

Procedure for Providing Hearing Protection

Step 1. Inform the client of the need for hearing protection. Be specific. For example, "You play in a rock band. In concerts and at practice, the sound levels you are exposed to will cause hearing loss."

Step 2. Obtain the client's agreement that he or she will wear hearing protection once fitted satisfactorily.

Step 3. Choose an ear-plug-type protector that is compatible with the client's needs.
   • A musician's ear plug capable of 15 dB of linear attenuation is available in a custom earmold.
   • Impact noise attenuators that attenuate the impact of gunfire but allow for conversation at normal conversational levels are available for shooters.
   • Exposure to high levels of continuous noise may be reduced by custom earplugs made of soft material, or by over-the-counter single, double, or triple flanged ear plugs.

Step 4. Orient the client to the ear plugs.
   • Show the client how to insert and remove the ear plugs. Observe the client seating and removing the ear plugs several times.
   • Inform the client of the need to reseat the ear plugs periodically while wearing them.
   • Inform the client that the ear plugs may be cleaned with mild soap and water.

Problem 6-14. The efficiency of the hearing conservation program is unknown.

Solution 6-14. Conduct a program analysis.

What is program efficiency? **Program efficiency** results from meeting program goals in a timely manner and utilizing only resources needed to accomplish the program's goals. Each component area of the hearing conservation program must be examined to determine whether the goals of that component were achieved in a timely manner without wasting program resources. The most time-consuming component of the hearing conservation program is identification audiometry. Therefore, it has the greatest potential to interfere with timely execution of the program as a whole.

When the definition of program efficiency is applied to the identification audiometry portion of the program, you realize that much can be done to increase efficiency. The person who is familiar with the equipment and the testing procedures obviously is much more efficient than the person who is not. Likewise, the person who has screened in the past will be faster. There are other less obvious examiner-related variables that affect the time needed to complete identification audiometry. Organization is one. Think about the screening situation. Are all of your movements efficient? Are all of your movements necessary? The more efficient the person doing the screening, the greater the time savings.

In addition to cooperative subjects and efficient testers, screening or testing protocols affect the total time spent in identification audiometry. Pure-tone screening takes less time than threshold testing. Pure-tone screening takes less time when the intensity is limited to a single level. Screening four frequencies per ear takes less time than screening six frequencies per ear. Screening pure-tone thresholds only takes less time than screening pure tones and immittance. This argument could be carried to the extreme. There is a point beyond which necessary information will be missed. Considerations of time and efficiency should not sacrifice the information needed to identify significant hearing problems.

Components of an Effective Hearing Conservation Program

From the discussion so far, it is apparent that hearing conservation programs contain several components—education, identification audiometry, reporting, and follow-up. We will now take a more detailed look at these and other components of an effective hearing conservation program.

Hearing conservation programs in all settings contain all or some of the following components:

- Noise survey
- Education

- Identification
- Follow-up
- Reporting
- Program evaluation.

Noise Survey

The noise survey component of a hearing conservation program involves measuring noise utilizing a sound level meter (SLM). There are two purposes for measuring noise:

- Specification of ambient noise levels for the determination of an acceptable test environment
- Specification of ambient noise levels for the determination of the acceptability of noise exposure.

General use of the SLM and noise measurement techniques may be covered in undergraduate coursework in audiology. Graduate courses in instrumentation, hearing conservation, and noise teach use of the SLM and noise evaluation techniques in greater detail. Speech-language pathologists who are using the SLM for the first time are able to learn enough from instrumentation manuals to become proficient at determining whether ambient noise levels are acceptable for screening. Graduate audiology students with course work in noise measurement are better able to measure excessive noise than are speech-language pathology students and beginning audiology students.

Specification of Ambient Noise Levels in the Test Environment

To answer the question, "Is the quiet area sufficiently quiet for hearing screening?" the allowable and existing levels of ambient noise must be compared. A mistake often made by the uninitiated is to assume that a quiet room is quiet enough for testing without making SLM measurements. Another mistake is to make measurements when the typical noises of changing classes, playground activities, equipment operation, and so forth are absent. Therefore, the first step is to make an accurate assessment of the ambient noise levels in the test environment.

Determine the Ambient Noise Levels in the Test Environment. The noise levels must be determined with an SLM. **Octave band** measurements are measurements of narrow bands of noise centered at octave intervals. These measurements must be made at times when the noise will represent actual ambient levels. The second step is to compare the measurements obtained with maximum allowable limits.

Allowable levels for hearing screening. Individuals must pass hearing screening at predetermined levels. If ambient noise levels exceed the predetermined screening level, individuals with normal hearing will fail the screening. **Ambient noise** is background noise from all sources that are in the test environment. Two factors must be considered when determining whether the level of ambient noise for hearing screening is sufficiently low:

- The sound pressure level (SPL) of noise that allows threshold testing to 0 dB Hearing Level (HL) under earphones and
- The predetermined screening level.

Table 6-1 presents the ambient noise level allowed to test threshold at 0 dB HL and the ambient noise level allowed for screening at 15 dB HL. Row 1 gives the SPL values by frequency of allowable noise to test hearing at 0 dB HL. These values represent normal human sensitivity in SPL plus the earphone cushion attenuation values. In row 2 of Table 6-1, the predetermined screening level of 15 dB is recorded. In row 3, the allowable limits of ambient room noise for your testing environment when screening at 15 dB HL is listed by octave band. To calculate ambient noise allowed for other screening levels, simply substitute that value into row 2 of Table 6-1 and add to the values in row 1.

When audiometers are equipped with earphone enclosures, greater levels of ambient noise can be tolerated. Earphone enclosures are miniature sound rooms that encase each earphone individually. Ear-

TABLE 6-1. Estimating allowable ambient noise levels (in dB SPL for octave bands) required to screen hearing at 15 dB HL.

CONDITION	FREQUENCY IN HERTZ						
	125	250	500	1000	2000	4000	8000
Under earphones	34.5	23.0	21.5	29.5	34.5	42.0	45.0
15 dB HL screening level	15	15	15	15	15	15	15
Total noise allowable	49.5	38.0	35.5	44.5	49.5	57.0	60.0

phone enclosures that seal properly against the side of the head may provide significant attenuation of ambient noise and enable screening to take place in an otherwise unacceptable environment. Earphone enclosures may be difficult to fit properly on smaller heads and can be uncomfortable. You do not need to use earphone enclosures unless they are required to provide sound treatment for a test environment with excessive ambient noise.

If your screening level is fixed and the ambient noise level is too great to allow screening at that level, alter the environment or find an acceptable environment. If this is not possible, do not screen. Screening under unacceptable ambient noise conditions will result in a high rate of false identification of hearing loss, because the noise levels in the test environment will mask out the test tone.

Specification of Ambient Noise Levels for Noise Exposure

Excessive noise may cause hearing loss, or it may interfere with tasks without endangering hearing. Audiology students in practicum may be expected to measure excessive noise in settings such as a manufacturing plant, an office, or a classroom.

One reason for identifying areas with excessive noise levels is to protect the hearing of the individuals in those areas from exposure to the noise. Excessive noise exposure depends on both noise level and time of exposure. **Time of exposure** refers to the amount of time the individual is in a noisy environment. It is important to obtain overall noise levels in dBA. Levels in dBA consider the threshold of sensitivity for the average normal-hearing ear. In addition to dBA measurements, it is important to obtain octave band measurements. Octave band measurement may reveal the cause of excessive noise.

Another type of excessive noise interferes with tasks. This type of noise may not exceed limits that are safe for hearing and, yet, be annoying. The noise may interfere with work that requires high levels of concentration. Some relatively low noise levels may cause headaches, irritation, and interference with communication. Management appreciates a happy and productive office and is open to suggestions to control unnecessary or annoying noise sources. Classrooms must have noise levels compatible with learning tasks. Bedrooms must be quiet enough to allow restful sleep. Kryter's (1985) book is an excellent reference source for documenting noise interference levels.

Education

Education most often is accomplished in three stages. In the first stage, an initial site visit is made and a conference with the administrator or an appointed representative is held to explain the purpose of the program and the program's components. A time is chosen to in-service the staff or supervisors and to conduct the testing. A procedure for educating the target population is decided on. A suitable testing environment is chosen at the initial site visit.

The initial meeting with the administrator is a two-way educational session. The administrator will be educated about program goals, procedures, and expected outcomes. The administrator will educate those in charge of executing the hearing conservation program about the facilities, those being served by the program, the staff, and the facility's schedule.

In the second phase, the actual in-service of staff or supervisory personnel is conducted. Teachers in the school, nurses in the nursing home, and supervisors in industry are examples of groups involved in this educational phase.

In the third phase, the target population is educated. School children may be taught about hearing and learn about dangers to hearing. Individual workers may be given information on reasons for hearing loss and methods of protecting hearing. Teachers may educate their classes about the hearing conservation program at their school and about protecting their hearing from loud noise. Staff physicians may educate workers with hearing loss about treatment options for existing loss and how to avoid additional hearing loss. The student in practicum also may be involved directly in this phase of educating the target population.

Education of administration or staff and the target population have different purposes. The purpose of educating administration and staff is to establish support for the program. The purpose of educating the target population is to create a positive attitude toward hearing conservation in those whose hearing is at risk. In different settings, administrators and personnel differ and the focus of the hearing conservation programs is different.

Identification

The identification audiometry component of a hearing conservation program involves screening or testing individuals at risk for hearing impairment. This component may utilize pure-tone audiometry, electrophysiologic testing, or a high-risk registry. The purpose of identification audiometry is to differentiate between individuals with hearing loss and those with normal hearing. Identification audiometry is setting specific and will be discussed in more detail in Chapters 7, 8, and 9.

Follow-Up Services

The follow-up component of a hearing conservation program involves providing treatment or referral services for individuals identified as at risk for hearing loss. An effective hearing conservation program cannot exist without an effective follow-up component.

Reporting

The reporting component of a hearing conservation program involves presenting background information, testing results, and recommendations. Reports serve as a record of service delivered and received. In addition, reports may serve public relations and marketing functions.

In some settings, the report on the hearing conservation program may be as simple as a listing of those who failed the screening. In other settings, great care is given to summarizing the program, stating criteria for referral, listing individuals tested and referred, and making specific recommendations for follow-up services.

There are advantages to thorough reporting. One obvious advantage is that it provides a record that can be used to check the effectiveness of follow-up services. A thorough record of a program also provides a basis for continuity for the program next year. A less obvious advantage is marketing. A thorough report makes a positive impression and will result in greater administrative support in future referrals.

The following sections are suggested for inclusion in a thorough report:

> • *An introduction.* The introduction should contain the name of the facility where the hearing conservation program was conducted and the name of the facility conducting the program, if different. The report should contain the inclusive dates when the program was conducted. It should state the purpose(s) of the program and list its major components. The report should mention all contact persons by name and date

and the content of the communication. It should mention in-services conducted, what was discussed, when they occurred, where they were held, and who attended.

* *A section on the criteria used in selecting the screening procedures.* The specific procedures used are stated in this section.
* *A data section.* This section should divide the screening data into a minimum of three categories: those screened, those absent and not screened, and those referred for further testing.
* *A recommendations section.* This is needed to explain the basis for specific referrals and to make those referrals.
* *A summary section.* This section is needed to state the number of people tested and the number referred. An estimation of the efficiency of the program in meeting its stated goals also should be included in this section.

Reports should be mailed with a cover letter to the facility administrator, thanking him or her for his or her cooperation, restating any additional follow-up commitments made, and setting an approximate date to initiate the next year's program.

Program Evaluation

The evaluation component of a hearing conservation program involves determining the effectiveness of the program. Without program evaluation, program quality cannot be measured or improved. In a thorough program evaluation, the service provider learns what was effective and what needs improvement. A few service providers ignore this component and miss opportunities to improve services and gain a competitive edge. Others conduct thorough but informal evaluations. A few conduct thorough formal evaluations.

One measure of the effectiveness of a hearing conservation program is how smoothly the program proceeded from initiation to completion. If the program was completed within the allotted time frame and met program objectives, it can be considered an effectively planned and executed program.

A measure of the effectiveness of the educational component of a hearing conservation program is the level of support provided by the administration and staff of the facility receiving the services. If administrators and staff were helpful and expressed pleasure with the service, the educational component can be considered effectively executed.

An identification program is effective when individuals with significant hearing problems are distinguished from those without such problems. One measure of that effectiveness occurs when individuals known to have hearing problems and those suspected of having hearing problems are identified. Likewise, an identification program is successful when only a few individuals referred as having hearing problems are not found to have hearing problems. A comparison between the results from identification audiometry and reports from referrals quickly reveals how many people identified as having hearing problems actually have hearing problems.

To determine how many individuals were identified as passing who should have been failed, a sample of those who passed the screening should be tested by a different tester or at a different facility. When the two sets of results are compared, a percentage of misidentifications can be ascertained. Unless the program meets an acceptable hit and miss rate in the identification component, the program cannot be considered effective, no matter how effective the other components of the program are.

Unless those identified as at risk for hearing impairment are followed and receive appropriate treatment, the hearing conservation program cannot receive high marks. What good does it do to identify hearing loss unless something is done about it? The follow-up component is effective when individuals at risk for hearing loss are monitored and receive treatment, as needed.

A reporting component is effective when all concerned can reconstruct the program from the report. A hearing conservation program may be effectively executed and followed up, but, unless it can be reconstructed and the data contained in the report, continuity is lost. Without a record, the next program offered must begin at ground zero and much needless repetition of effort will occur.

Unless a thorough evaluation of the hearing conservation program occurs, it is difficult to know whether the activity is worthwhile. Even if the supervisor or facility at which the student is in practicum does not require an evaluation of the hearing conservation program, the student must complete an evaluation of the effectiveness of the program to know what was learned by participating in it.

Settings for Hearing Conservation Programs

All hearing conservation programs have common goals. Many have common components, but there are important differences to consider between programs aimed at various populations in different settings. The student in practicum should be aware of these differences so that the hearing conservation program in which the student is involved has all the necessary components. Settings in which hearing conservation programs are implemented include the:

- school
- community
- workplace

Chapters 7, 8, and 9 present information specific to each setting, organized under program components headings.

7
The School Setting

School hearing conservation programs usually are discussed in introductory courses in audiology. Most states mandate public school hearing conservation programs. Although there may be differences from state to state, these programs contain many common components. Public school nurses typically are in charge of administering hearing conservation programs. Even in public schools that hire educational audiologists, the school nurse most often screens children's hearing. The educational audiologist may administer follow-up testing for children referred from the screening and provide services for children with hearing problems.

Because they do not receive state monies, private schools are not required to offer hearing conservation programs mandated for public schools. However, private schools may provide hearing conservation programs as a service to their students. Clinics that offer audiologic services may offer hearing conservation services for private schools as a means of providing community service and of marketing their clinic services.

Hearing loss may interfere with children's speech, language, and learning development or indicate hearing health problems. Studies have shown that children with hearing losses greater than 15 dB HL perform significantly more poorly in school than children with better hearing

(Davis, Elfenbein, Schum, & Bentler, 1986; Quigley, 1968; Ross & Giolas, 1978).

Compared to older children and adults, preschool- and early elementary school-age children have a higher incidence of middle ear problems. Middle ear infection can progress into more serious health problems. It should be identified and, when appropriate, treated. From then on, the child's hearing should be monitored regularly. In addition to a having a higher incidence of middle ear disease, children may be exposed to excessive noise or ototoxins that may result in progressive high-frequency hearing loss. Some cultural groups in various areas of the country celebrate many social events with fireworks. As a result, it is not uncommon to see noise trauma notches in young children's audiograms.

Many state regulations for public school hearing conservation programs stipulate screening of children's hearing in kindergarten or first grade, third grade, fifth grade, and every third year thereafter. For the program conducted annually, these are appropriate grade levels to screen.

Screenings usually are conducted at a specific intensity level and at specific frequencies. State laws mandate intensity levels and specific frequencies to be screened for public schools. The student in practicum should obtain copies of and become familiar with state laws and ASHA guidelines pertaining to hearing screening of school children. Some private school hearing screening programs simply follow the standards for intensity and frequency specified for the public schools by state law.

Some states provide manuals that summarize state requirements. To receive a copy of the information available from your state, contact the state hearing conservation specialist in the Department of Health. Some manuals are very brief. Other manuals are designed to be used as course texts for training audiometric technicians to conduct public school hearing conservation programs. Some of these manuals provide helpful suggestions, examples of forms, and other useful information.

Ideally, to detect potential hearing problems that may cause learning difficulties early in the school year, hearing screening should be done in mid-September to mid-October. However, practicum assignments are usually made for a semester or quarter at a time. University training programs that expect all their practicum students to participate in school screening must schedule screening programs throughout the school year. Therefore, hearing screenings may identify children with significant hearing problems late in the school year. When this occurs, follow-up becomes even more important to ensure that the student receives needed services.

A problem that is identified late may result in the realization on the part of the school administration, teachers, and parents that better service is possible. Be aware that a problem discovered late is better than a problem undiscovered. Many of the schools with which you will be involved would not have any hearing conservation program unless provided later in the school year.

In the school setting, days when assemblies and other special programs are scheduled should be avoided when scheduling hearing screening. Elementary students, in particular, often require a day to settle into the school routine and are distracted on the last day of the week in anticipation of the weekend. The best days of the week to schedule hearing screening are Tuesday through Thursday when no special activities are planned.

The time of day when screenings are conducted also is important. Many kindergarten classes are half day. Some schools have a morning class and an afternoon class. If the facility has preschool children, there are scheduled napping times. Some schools open each day with an assembly or chapel program. Hearing screenings should begin after daily opening exercises and not interfere with lunch and nap times. Children should not be kept after the regular school day. If possible, screenings are best scheduled between 9:00 A.M. and 12:00 noon and between 1:00 P.M. and 2:30 P.M.

Noise Survey

The noise survey component of the school hearing conservation program involves two activities:

- Evaluating the test environment
- Identifying excessive noise

Evaluating Test Environment

Most public and private schools do not have special environments designed for screening hearing. Therefore, designated quiet areas are set aside temporarily for screening hearing. SLM measurements must be made to determine whether ambient noise levels in the designated area are acceptable for screening hearing.

Identifying Excessive Noise

There are environments in schools that produce excessive noise levels. Junior and senior high school programs often include wood and metal working shops, automotive repair shops, and other activities that produce excessive noise levels. The administrative staff of an educational facility should be questioned regarding activities that generate loud noise levels. Once sources of possible excessive noise levels are identified, measurements can be taken. Measurements should be taken at the position of the exposed ear(s) and the duration of the exposure should be determined. Students in schools are seldom exposed to an equivalent level of 85 dBA for an 8-hour day. However, staff may be. Even if no one is exposed to excessive and somewhat constant noise levels, taking noise measurements of possible offending areas provides an opportunity to educate persons working in those areas to the hazards of noise exposure.

Education

In addition to educating administrative staff, teachers and students should be educated about hearing conservation. Teachers are a great resource in preparing their students to be screened. Therefore, care should be taken to enlist their active participation in the program. In-service for teachers and administrators should take place a week or two before the screening so that teachers have time to prepare themselves and their students for screening without unduly interrupting previously scheduled class activities. Teachers often prepare class rosters and name tags for screening.

Teachers, administrators and, separately, students should be offered general information on the anatomy and physiology of the hearing system. This background information is necessary to explain the types of hearing loss. Information on types of hearing loss should be offered to explain the effects that noise, impacted ear wax, and middle ear problems have on hearing. With teachers and administrators, treatment options for common disorders may be discussed. In the separate session with the students, some very general and nonthreatening information regarding treatment for ear wax and middle ear effusion may be presented, if brought up by the students. For example, one might say, "ear wax can be cleaned out of the ear. Audiologists or physicians do it because they have a light that lets them see inside the ear." An example of what one might say about treatment for middle ear effusion is, "It often happens with colds and the medicine for the cold often clears up the middle ear problems."

The clinician should not bring up surgery. Often there is a child who has experienced tube placement. If the child brings it up, the clinician should reassure the other children that tubes are used as a last resort for someone whose hearing problems did not respond to medication. The clinician should not to frighten children with the possibility that participation in the program will result in surgery.

Information about protecting hearing from excessive noise should be emphasized. The detrimental effects of rock concerts, shooting, fireworks, and the noisy workplace should be specifically discussed.

Once information about hearing loss, its prevention, and treatment has been presented, information regarding the identification component of the program can be presented and screening techniques demonstrated. As stated before, screening time depends on a cooperative child. A child's cooperation may be better ensured with the proper preparation. The person conducting the educational session should explain the procedure and its purpose.

Terms such as "test," "fail," and "hearing loss" should be avoided in the explanation. Students should be allowed to try on a pair of earphones in the safe and familiar surroundings of their classrooms. Students who are apprehensive should be encouraged to go to the screening area to check it out for themselves on the day of the screening. Finally, time for the children to ask questions and make comments must be allowed.

Students in practicum may not count hours of staff in-service as clinical contact. Educating children who are to be screened may be counted as counseling. After appropriate education of the children, the identification component begins.

Identification

Identification audiometry in the school setting usually consists of pure-tone screening of several frequencies for each ear at a set intensity level. Some programs also include otoscopy and immittance audiometry to screen for middle ear problems.

There are several effective ways to coordinate the movement of students to and from the screening area. An effective method is to begin with one class and have the teacher of that class, or the teacher's designee, notify the next class when they are finished.

The teacher or his or her aide may supervise the children waiting to be screened and return those who have been screened to their classrooms. If the number of waiting students is small, it may be good to have the students wait in the screening area and observe the screening of their classmates. This procedure works well to familiarize younger students with the procedure and allay their concerns. Reluctant students can be passed over until they are comfortable with the screening process.

Name tags pinned to students' clothing ensures correct spelling of names and provides a cross-check for who has been screened. When the student presents for screening, the name tag should be removed by the person doing the screening. In the school setting, students have been known to have been screened and returned to the end of the line to be screened again. Reasons for this behavior vary from "this is more fun than class" to "I didn't know what else to do." Duplicate screening can be avoided with name tags.

Some facilities utilize immittance equipment when screening preschool and early elementary school-age children. Immittance audiometry picks up middle ear conditions that may be missed in puretone screening. If immittance equipment is used, it must be properly calibrated before and at intervals during the testing. Immittance testing also requires a method of cleaning ear tips. If ear tips are the insert type, an otoscope and tweezers are necessary. The student clinician is expected to be familiar with equipment and screening procedures. Most of this information is provided in introductory course work in audiology.

The time needed to screen the hearing of a child varies with the cooperativeness of the child, the amount of screening to be done, and the organization, skill, and confidence of the tester. If the child is cooperative, the tester competent, and the screening limited to pure tones, total screening time will be under 2 minutes.

Two of the factors that influence the intensity levels and frequencies chosen for screening are:

- The criteria for hearing
- The ambient noise levels

Many state-mandated hearing screening levels are 25 dB HL. ASHA suggests 20 dB HL. A 15 dB HL screening level may be preferable for school children. Learning new tasks in a primarily oral-aural environment requires sensitive hearing. A child with a hearing level of 15 dB HL may be a candidate for amplification in the classroom. However 15 dB HL screening level is possible only when ambient noise levels in the testing environment allow it.

In many school settings, ambient noise levels will not allow screening, even with earphone enclosures, at 15 dB HL. However, screening at 20 or 25 dB HL may be possible. Ambient noise levels in school settings are primarily low frequency. Screening may be possible at 25 dB HL at 500 Hz and 15 dB HL at 1000 Hz through 8000 Hz. You must use the noise survey information for the testing environment to determine appropriate screening levels.

The number of frequencies screened depends on program goals. The frequency spectrum of 300 to 3000 Hz includes most important speech information. It follows that a child may be able to hear quite well for learning with a modified frequency range. Screening may be limited to 500, 1000, 2000, and 3000 or 4000 Hz. To identify more children with noise trauma, it is wise to add 6000 Hz. When program goals can be met with fewer frequencies screened and ambient noise problems can be avoided by testing fewer frequencies, it makes sense to limit the frequencies tested.

Identification of significant middle-ear problems may be an additional goal in a hearing screening program. Three methods are more effective than pure-tone air conduction screening. Otoscopic examination and immittance screening are the two most common techniques used. A third technique is to utilize a bone vibrator, with the ears unoccluded, placed on either mastoid and present a 500 Hz tone at 5 dB HL. If the child responds to the tone, there is a good chance that a significant conductive hearing loss is keeping ambient noise from reaching the child's inner ear. This method of screening for conductive hearing loss requires an audiometer with bone-conduction test capability. All three techniques can meet the goal of identifying middle ear problems missed by pure-tone testing.

Children should not be forced to have their hearing screened. However, neither should a child be given permission to reject the screening. Parents may withhold permission for their children to be screened, but children should not be placed in the position of controlling whether or not they are screened. Parents and teachers who are properly prepared are more likely to present cooperative children.

One of the authors (BRK) has experienced several situations which demonstrate the importance of parents and teachers in the child's spirit of cooperativeness. For example, one teacher explained the procedure as a *test* that the kindergartners would either pass or fail and compared having their hearing screened to a visit to the doctor's office. When several children expressed anxiety, the class was told that they had no choice but to be tested. When that class came to the screening area, the teacher pushed one child forward and said, "You have had your hearing tested before. Show the others how it is done." The child began to cry. The class began to cry. With great care and much time, the screener was able to turn the situation around and accomplish the screening. It took 2 hours to screen 20 children.

On the same occasion, while the screening was being conducted, one mother marched her kindergartner in late and announced, "I want Sally's hearing screened, but she probably will not let you test her. She thinks all doctors hurt!" Needless to say, Sally did not let anyone screen her hearing.

There are numerous examples of sensitive and well-prepared teachers whose students look forward to the screening as an adventure. To maintain their positive and cooperative attitudes, the screener should be friendly, nonthreatening, and firm. Kneel down to the child's level. Smile. Instruct simply. Confirm that the child understands the task and what his or her response is to be.

Never ask the child's permission to do any part of the screening procedure. If you ask if you can place the earphones and the child says no, you will have to honor the child's decision. The child will not be screened. Be careful using the phrase "okay," as in "I am going to place the earphones on your head now, okay?" The child may interpret "okay" as a question to which he or she can say "no." A child is seldom uncooperative without reason. Do not provide a child with reason to be uncooperative.

It also is important to prepare those to be screened properly for the experience. Relate to the children being screened in a positive, friendly, and competent manner, and allow children to be screened an opportunity to observe others being screened. If a child expresses reluctance to participate in the screening, reseat him or her with the children observing the screening. Allow the child to watch several more screenings and then try again. Often children will be ready after observing a few more classmates complete the procedure. If not, reseat them with those observing and try again later. If all else fails, use firm but friendly coaxing to screen the child. However, a child who remains uncooperative at this point should be recorded as not testable and returned to the classroom.

In addition to the child's cooperativeness, screening time depends on the screener's competence. There are subtle examiner-related variables that affect screening time. Organization is one. If the screener presents the tone in the right ear at 500, 1000, 2000, and 4000 Hz, switches to the left ear and presents the tone at 4000, 2000, 1000, and 500 Hz, the screening time will be shorter than if the examiner switched back to 500 Hz when beginning the left ear. Use of a form listing students' names by class that can be checked off is more efficient than hand writing the names of children as they are tested. Think about the screening situation. The more efficient the person doing the screening is, the greater the amount of time saved.

In addition to cooperative students and efficient screeners, the screening protocol affects screening time. Screening four frequencies per ear takes less time than screening six frequencies per ear. Screening only pure-tone thresholds takes less time than screening pure tones and immittance.

Reporting

Great care should be taken to summarize the hearing conservation program in the school setting. The report should include all criteria used, including those for referral. The report should list those tested and children referred and make specific recommendations for follow-up services.

Reports should be mailed with a cover letter to the school administrator. In this letter, the clinician should thank the administrator for his or her cooperation, restate any additional follow-up commitments made, and set an approximate date to initiate the next year's program.

Follow-up Services

The purpose of identifying children with hearing problems is to make parents aware of their needs and to recommend treatment. If the parent is aware of the child's problems, it is important to know if the child is being managed currently. A few well-chosen questions about current medications and the child's next scheduled visit to the doctor will help evaluate whether the child is being actively managed. Make notes and include this information in your report. If a child currently under audiologic or medical management fails the screening, the managing specialist should be notified.

Children who fail the pure-tone screening should be referred for diagnostic audiology. If a child is suspected of having a conductive involvement and is not currently under audiologic, medical, or both kinds of management, the child should be referred for diagnostic audiology. Serial immittance audiometry often is required to plot recovery from middle ear problems.

The school may insist on taking the entire responsibility for follow-up services. Schools often control communication to the parents so that confusion and misinterpretation are held to a minimum. However, personal telephone contact between the person in charge of the screening and the parents enables the parents to schedule appointments, ask questions, or give pertinent information. For example, a child identified as being at risk may already be under medical care for middle ear infection.

Follow-up on individual students should begin immediately after the submission of the report to the school, if the follow-up protocol has been approved by the school. After completion of the follow-up component of the hearing conservation program, the information generated by the program is available for evaluation.

Program Evaluation

In evaluating of the effectiveness of a school hearing conservation program, the following questions must be answered:

- Were program goals met in a timely fashion?
- Were program resources utilized efficiently?

It is important to understand the criteria used in a school hearing conservation program and each component within the program and to ensure that those involved in the program understand the criteria. Often criteria are not stated, but assumed from screening levels, or criteria may emphasize only positive goals and ignore program limitations.

Unless program limitations are explained to school personnel and to parents, they often assume that all children who pass the screening have normal hearing. Such an assumption invalidates the entire hearing conservation program. If ambient noise levels prevent screening at levels below 25 dB HL, most children with impacted wax and active middle ear effusion will be missed. Children who have normal hearing on the day of the test may develop hearing problems at a later date. When parents and school personnel assume that passing a screening test on Tuesday protects a child from developing significant hearing problems on Wednesday, hearing conservation efforts may be undermined. Parents and school personnel need to be made aware that hearing health requires constant vigilance.

Program criteria must be consistent with identification audiometry. Program limitations must be emphasized to avoid establishing false expectations in school personnel, parents, and students. If program criteria, stated or otherwise, result in false expectations regarding any aspect of hearing conservation program, it has been a disservice to the community.

Services that create a false impression that hearing has been adequately tested when it has not may prevent individuals from seeking services when they are needed. It is not true that some services are better than no services at all.

In addition to program criteria, the effectiveness of the identification audiometry needs to be evaluated. In identification audiometry errors are inevitable. The question is: "How much error do we accept and of what type?" A rule of thumb is that the person screening should produce the same results as a trained, experienced tester 90% of the time. A rule of thumb regarding acceptable error is that no more than 5% of those with hearing loss should be missed and no more than 5% of those with normal hearing should be falsely identified as having hearing problems. One procedure by which the efficiency of the identification component can be ascertained is to have the supervisor rescreen every 10th child, creating a sample from which program efficiency can be derived.

A hearing conservation program may have appropriate and well-understood criteria. It may have an efficient screening component. However, unless follow-up in the form of appropriate diagnosis and treatment happens, the program is neither efficient nor effective. One method of evaluating the efficiency of the follow-up component of the hearing conservation program is to interview the parents of children referred for follow-up services within 6 weeks after the screening.

Often the student in practicum is assigned this task. When telephoning parents, identify yourself and what you are calling about. Restate the recommendation made for their child and politely inquire regarding their follow-up.

If the child who was referred was found to have no problems on referral, be prepared for a parent who may harbor some hostility. Be sure to inform the parent that a small number of referral errors do occur and apologize for any inconvenience that may have resulted. Also, be aware that some problems identified by screening may resolve themselves prior to the child being seen for treatment.

8

Community Settings

C ommunity hearing conservation programs can be divided into three types:

- Health fairs
- Senior citizen settings
- Neonatal hospital facilities

Health Fairs

Some hearing conservation programs are designed to offer a community service and to market clinic services. These may be conducted in university and hospital clinic facilities, at community centers, area health fairs held in auditoriums, and open or enclosed shopping malls. Because hearing screening is offered free and nothing is being sold, no laws specify the components of this service. The primary goals of community hearing conservation programs are to educate the general public about hearing, hearing conservation, and hearing loss. A secondary goal is to generate clinical referrals.

Hearing is necessary for effective communication, and communication becomes more and more important to people as they grow older.

When persons retire, their lives are built around their relationships, family, and friends. Relationships are maintained through communication. When they are unable to hear, many older persons withdraw from communication and, as a result, lose out on social interaction. Their quality of life is diminished.

Hearing conservation programs in community settings can be grouped into two general categories:

- Specific programs
- General community programs

Specific programs may be related to issues of zoning for noise control. Many cities have zoning codes restricting noise above specified levels at different times during the 24-hour day. For example, the overflight of residential areas by aircraft is regulated. Noise levels from vehicular traffic also may be regulated.

Specific programs may be related to recreational activities, hobbies, or leisure time activities. Some forms of recreation produce hazardous noise levels. For example, rock concerts often produce potentially hazardous noise levels. Using a chain saw to cut wood produces hazardous noise levels. Other examples of activities that produce noise levels hazardous to hearing are snowmobiling, model airplane building and flying, shooting, hunting, wood and metal working, lawn mowing, and using power tools at home.

The purpose of hearing conservation programs related to specific activities is to reduce risk of damage to hearing by educating those involved in the activities and to identify hearing loss in the populations involved in the activities. Most hearing conservation activities to date in these areas have consisted of limited educational activities, such as articles in trade magazines.

A person who experiences hearing loss attributable to specific activities often will seek professional diagnosis and treatment. When the audiologist identifies such a person, the person will receive individualized education and treatment. Practicum students should be aware of opportunities to educate clients regarding the hazards of recreational noise.

Community hearing conservation is important. Many people involved in activities that are hazardous to their hearing are not exposed to hearing conservation programs in the workplace or school. Therefore, they are often unaware of the danger of noise exposure. Hearing loss is insidious. It occurs gradually and often is experienced as a loss of clarity in hearing before overall hearing levels are reduced to the point that hearing loss is suspected.

Community hearing conservation programs, especially those connected with community health fairs, may become annual affairs. Many times they are one-time events. Community hearing conservation programs are continued when well thought-out and executed programs result in effective community education and clinical referrals.

Community hearing conservation programs often are held in conjunction with other community events or as a part of community health fairs. Such events are usually scheduled on days and at times accessible to the general working public.

With the community hearing conservation program, the potential client base is generated by pre-event advertising. Community calendar announcements through the media are effective, as are other advertising channels.

Noise Surveys

When participating in community health fairs and other events to promote hearing services and hearing conservation, hearing screening is a primary activity. Hearing screening provides an opportunity to discuss concerns the people being screened might have regarding their hearing. The screening environments at such events (indoor or outdoor malls, a gymnasium, etc.) have high ambient noise levels and may also be highly reverberant. In a highly reverberant room, noise bounces around. Hearing screening conducted in such an environment can be highly suspect. It is imperative that an accurate estimation of ambient noise levels be made. Ambient noise at such frequencies as 3000 Hz or 4000 Hz may allow screening at an acceptable level of 30 to 35 dB HL. You do not know until you measure it using a sound level meter and an octave band analyzer.

Sometimes students in practicum are involved in measuring noise levels in the community for reasons other than determining whether ambient noise levels in test areas are acceptable. Noise measurements are conducted when complaints of noise result in litigation. Also, such measurements are made when questions arise during litigation concerning a person's ability to hear. It is possible for the audiology student in practicum who is majoring in audiology to serve as an assistant to a licensed audiologist and be involved in noise measurements of this type. Because many of these situations result in or from litigation and require credentials as an expert witness, it would be unethical for a student in practicum to accept primary responsibility for these measurements. Again, Kryter (1985) has provided an excellent resource for noise measurement.

Education

In the general community setting, the educational component is conducted one-on-one. Therefore, community hearing conservation programs often involve a great deal of informational counseling and counseling dealing with feelings and attitudes. There is often little privacy possible when counseling in a community hearing conservation program. Effective counseling of individuals with hearing loss requires an academic background in counseling and management of individuals with hearing loss. Also, closely supervised experience in counseling and management of individuals with hearing loss is desirable before the student in practicum is ready for the educational component of the community hearing conservation experience. First semester practicum students often are relegated to screening hearing while an audiologist counsels the individuals screened about their results.

The persons in charge of the community hearing conservation program are responsible for the flow of recipients of the service through the program. There is no third party, like the teacher in the school hearing conservation program in charge of a group of participants coming through. There is only the individual and his or her family who are requesting information. Education about hearing, possible hearing loss, hearing evaluation, and management of hearing loss is the most important aspect of this type of community hearing conservation program. The targets of this education are the individuals seeking information and the significant others with them.

Identification

In the community hearing conservation program, there may be no coordination of movement of preselected groups to a testing facility or area. The individuals who receive services may be persons who are drawn by pre-event advertising or simply are passing by. It is important for the area in which the hearing conservation program is offered to be in the main flow of traffic. The area should look inviting and entice people to stop and talk.

In the community hearing conservation program, screening is offered rather than required. All those who stop by the screening area, who accept the offer to have their hearing screened, are screened. First semester practicum students can administer the screening.

Even though audiometric screening or threshold testing is usually a component of hearing conservation programs, it is often not the primary emphasis in the general community hearing conservation effort. In fact, the acoustic environment may be so poor that hearing screening is almost impossible to conduct, and the results obtained must be interpreted cautiously. This is not to say that screening audiometry under these conditions should be discouraged, only that results must be interpreted with appropriate qualification.

Screening should be conducted in the same area where initial contact is made and where counseling takes place. Equipment and personnel conducting the screening should be far enough apart to give the appearance of a minimal level of sound control and confidentiality.

At a well-attended health fair, a steady stream of interested individuals can be handled adequately by two persons screening without creating a waiting line. If the hearing conservation area is inundated with persons, it is best to abbreviate procedures to move people through faster. If waiting becomes necessary, a half dozen folding chairs is usually sufficient. A line of more than four or five people can be encouraged to visit other areas and to return in a few minutes when the line thins out. It is very important to keep waiting time to a minimum.

Portable pure-tone audiometers are versatile equipment for audiology programs and services. They are readily available for hearing conservation programs, including community hearing conservation programs.

Practicum students should have a supervisor who holds CCC-A available to them at all times. An audiologist involved in counseling cannot really be considered available for supervision of practicum students unless he or she observes the students screening prior to counseling the individual being screened.

Adults are the largest population presenting themselves for hearing screening in community hearing conservation programs. The intensity level and the number of frequencies screened are entirely dependent on ambient noise levels and program criteria. When program criteria are to identify high-frequency sensorineural hearing loss in an environment with high levels of low-frequency ambient noise, screening at 35 dB HL at 3000 Hz may be appropriate. A large proportion of adults with significant hearing loss will be identified.

Reporting

In the general community setting, the hearing conservation service often is initiated by a clinical program. There may be no organization to whom the results would be reported. However, maintaining a written report on the activities, including the names and addresses of potential clients, is a good idea. From such a report, follow-up services can be initiated. In addition, a record is available to provide information on what was effective and what was not. What was effective may be used again. What was not effective may be eliminated.

A short in-house report is appropriate for community hearing conservation programs. The audiologist in charge may prefer to compile the report. A better practicum experience would assign that responsibility to a student. Information that needs to be reported includes:

- program criteria
- number of persons contacted
- number of persons screened and counseled
- number of referrals made.

Follow-Up Services

It is important to obtain names, addresses, and telephone numbers of each person referred. From that information, persons can be contacted and scheduled. Follow-up on the individual then becomes a part of regularly scheduled clinical follow-up services.

The program conducting the community hearing conservation program should refer all individuals needing services to the clinical facility providing the service. To generate the referrals and then to refer them elsewhere is counterproductive.

Telephone surveys are appropriate follow-up tools. Some surveys of this type include several specific yes/no questions which the caller is to read and check an answer. The questions may include:

1. Was your hearing screened?
2. Do you have hearing loss?
3. Does your hearing loss cause you problems?
4. What treatment is available for your loss?
5. Do you plan to seek treatment?
6. May I schedule you?
7. Would you refer family members, friends, or acquaintances for hearing testing?

Program Evaluation

Evaluation of a community hearing conservation program should determine whether the program achieved its goals of increasing public awareness of hearing conservation and generating clinical referrals. One way to evaluate whether the program increased participant awareness of hearing and hearing conservation is through telephone interviews. The caller should identify him- or herself and the purpose of the call. The person called should be asked what he or she learned from the program. Again, persons who are screened should realize that screening is not diagnostic testing.

The success of the hearing conservation program in generating referrals can be tracked by noting if clients referred by the program presented for services. Not all referrals come in immediately following the date they were referred. To evaluate the effectiveness of the program, data should be recorded over a period of several months.

The Senior Citizen Setting

Hearing conservation programs for the senior citizen most often are conducted in senior citizen community centers, retirement homes, and nursing homes. The populations in these settings differ greatly, and the hearing conservation programs must be adapted accordingly.

Even though there are no laws, ASHA position papers and guidelines regulating the delivery of hearing conservation services in senior settings, examples of effective programs, and discussions of issues related to conserving the hearing of senior citizens have been published in various professional journals to assist the professional and the student in practicum in delivering quality services. In any case, professional audiologists, clinic supervisors, and student clinicians are bound by professional ethics.

Hearing loss and hearing handicap need to be differentiated. The medico-legal definition for normal hearing is better than 25 dB HL for the frequencies 250 Hz through 8000 Hz. Therefore, **hearing loss** is hearing worse than 25 dB HL. **Hearing handicap** results when hearing loss interferes with or causes an individual to alter his or her life style. Hearing handicap is a separate variable to be addressed after hearing loss has been identified.

Seniors with hearing losses greater than 25 dB HL may have difficulty hearing well enough to communicate effectively. For example, instructions regarding medication may not be heard correctly.

Significant hearing loss affects one of three persons above age 65. The more advanced age groups have greater incidence of hearing loss.

Senior citizens have a higher incidence of sensorineural hearing loss than younger individuals. However, wax impaction and resulting conductive hearing problems are also quite common. These problems should be identified, treated if appropriate, and the person's hearing monitored on a regular basis.

Hearing should be screened annually. It is prudent to screen all residents. If not, many with hearing problems may be missed. However, it must be remembered that screening programs offered in senior citizens' facilities are voluntary, and many seniors may choose not to be involved.

The mentally alert elderly person may be able to function with mild hearing loss. Important factors to consider in determining hearing handicap are situational listening demands, level of activity, attitude, relative independence, and family support. If a person's waking time is spent sitting alone in front of the television, the situational listening demands and level of activity are not high. Turning the television volume up to compensate for a mild hearing loss may disturb no one and provide the individual with the needed amplification. When the hearing loss borders on moderate or the senior's life style demands better hearing, treatment for the hearing loss becomes necessary.

Noise Survey

Screening the hearing of senior citizens may take place in community senior citizens' facilities, senior citizens' retirement facilities, or nursing homes. In some of these facilities, areas with acceptable ambient noise levels are available. Others have high ambient noise levels in highly reverberant fields. Therefore, ambient noise conditions in the area to be used for screening should be measured under the conditions in which the screening is to be conducted. Again, in high ambient noise frequencies such as 3000 Hz or 4000 Hz may allow screening at an acceptable level of 30 to 35 dB HL. Without the use of a sound level meter and an octave band analyzer, ambient levels can only be guessed.

Education

There are parallels to be drawn between educational components of hearing conservation programs in schools and senior citizen settings.

Education in the senior citizen setting is most often accomplished in two stages. In the first stage, an initial site visit is made to explain the program and plan for its implementation.

In the second stage, education of staff is accomplished, usually within the time frame of a scheduled staff meeting. In some nursing care facilities staff may be divided into two to three shifts. The number of staff meetings may be reduced by meeting between two shifts.

You should allow 15 to 20 minutes for presentation and 5 minutes for questions. The surroundings in which the inservice is conducted should encourage interaction. Staff are a great resource in preparing residents to be screened, and great care should be taken to enlist their active participation in the program.

Identification

As in schools and general community settings, identification audiometry in the senior citizen setting is screening rather than testing. A draft for peer review of a document presenting guidelines for the identification of hearing impairment and handicap in adult elderly persons appeared in *Asha* (ASHA Subcommittee, 1989). However, as of July, 1992, screening levels and frequencies for use with seniors had not been suggested by an offical ASHA position statement. Service providers must choose levels and frequencies that make sense in their individual programs.

Intensity levels used for screening with senior citizens have varied from threshold screening to 40 dB HL. When the hearing conservation service provides amplification as part of its follow-up services, threshold screening, as opposed to 25 dB HL, is often the method of identification audiometry. When follow-up services consist of referral for audiologic diagnostic testing, screening at a single frequency at 35 dB may be the method of choice. Most often, identification audiometry in the senior citizen setting consists of screening several frequencies at 25 dB HL.

Frequencies chosen for screening have varied from a single frequency of 2000 or 3000 Hz to multiple frequencies per ear. Common practice has been to screen 250 through 6000 Hz per ear in an attempt to identify low- as well as high-frequency hearing problems. Ambient noise levels may limit the frequencies that can be meaningfully screened. It is recommended that hearing be screened at 25 dB HL for the frequencies of 500, 1000, 2000, 4000 Hz in both ears.

There are several effective ways to coordinate the movement of individuals to and from the screening area. It is especially important to allow the administrator and front office input in how residents move to cause as little disruption as possible. It may be most appropriate for the section nurse to deliver his or her patients in the nursing home environment. It also may be appropriate to go to a resident's living area. For residents who are neurologically involved, name tags pinned to their clothing ensures correct spelling of names and provide a cross-check for who has been screened. Whatever system of moving residents to the screening area or the screening to the residents is chosen, it is important to create an even flow of residents to be screened.

In residential senior citizen facilities, there are not necessarily particular days of the week that are better to schedule hearing screening. The time needed to screen the hearing of a senior adult varies. If the person is cooperative, the tester competent, and the screening limited to the octave intervals between and including 500 Hz and 4000 Hz at a single intensity level, total screening time will be under 5 minutes. Often senior adults, especially those in nursing homes, are lonely. They are likely to engage the screener in conversation which can extend the testing time significantly. You should be prepared either to devote more time per individual during the screening process or to practice your skill at disengaging without offending.

The student in practicum should be aware that seniors in different settings present with different levels of difficulty in understanding and following directions. In senior citizen centers and residential settings, the majority of the seniors are alert, active adults, and present few special problems.

In the nursing home, residents are often ill, and may be angry, disoriented, or neurologically involved. Nursing home residents are seldom intentionally uncooperative, but that does happen, too. Residents in nursing homes often require a great deal of patience and a significantly longer time to screen. With these individuals, the person screening must be ready to accept limited data or to abort screening. However, the student in practicum should muster all of his or her people-skills to obtain complete screenings on all those presented for screening, if possible. The student should not be afraid to request assistance from the supervisor. Much learning in practicum is situation specific and can be demonstrated most effectively in individual settings.

As a general rule of thumb, older senior citizens have slower reaction times than do younger seniors. Be careful not to rush tone presentations to the point that the individual being screened becomes confused. Also, when tone presentations are rushed, the examiner may confuse a response to one presentation when it is actually to another.

Reporting

As stated earlier, there are advantages to thorough reporting. The hearing conservation program in the senior citizen setting should be an ongoing program. Therefore, quarterly reports to the administration are a good technique for keeping the program visible to the administration. Quarterly reports also are useful for stimulating regular program review.

Follow-Up Services

Some programs recommend that individuals identified as having hearing loss be brought to the clinical facility for diagnostic testing. Other programs deliver many of the services needed at the senior setting. Whatever the appropriate follow-up, it should take place as soon as the individual at risk for hearing problems is identified.

The purpose of identifying senior citizens with hearing problems is to make individuals and their significant others aware of their needs and to recommend management. If individuals are aware of their problems, it is important to know if they are being managed currently. Make notes and include this information in your report. To know what treatment is appropriate, diagnostic audiologic testing is often needed. Individuals who fail the pure-tone screening should be referred for diagnostic audiology. If follow-up testing for those referred by the program is not rendered at the facility, outside referrals should be made to audiologic and medical offices in the geographic service area.

As in the school setting, the senior facility may insist on taking the entire responsibility for follow-up services. They often control the communication with significant others so that confusion and misinterpretation are held to a minimum. However, personal telephone contact between the person in charge of the screening and the significant others enables appointments to be scheduled, questions to be asked, or pertinent information to be given.

Program Evaluation

In the senior citizen setting, the efficiency of the program is related to the number of people on staff and seniors who are more aware of hearing loss and its effects on communication. A systematic sampling of program participants can provide this information.

It is important to assess whether the participants identified as having a hearing loss have sought treatment. In a follow-up survey, individuals referred may be asked whether they have sought treatment, with whom, and of what type. Again, be sure that all individuals are aware that screening is not diagnostic testing.

To evaluate whether the hearing conservation program in the senior center generated referrals, clinic records may be examined. Careful record keeping on referral sources for clients seen will reveal the number of clients generated by the hearing conservation program.

The Neonatal Setting

Another special case of community hearing conservation occurs with the screening of neonates in the hospital setting. **Neonatal** designates the first 28 days of life. Few such programs exist in hospitals in the United States at this time because of limited resources. However, a few programs exist, some are funded from grants and administered in conjunction with university training programs. In these programs, the student has a valuable practicum opportunity with neonates.

Identification and follow-up of neonates at risk for hearing loss are important. Hearing loss that interferes with the development of communication skills and learning and hearing loss that indicates hearing health problems are more effectively treated when they are identified early. Greater numbers of neonates in intensive care units are affected than in well baby units. Overall, significant hearing loss affects 4% of neonates.

In many hospitals today, well babies and new mothers are released within 12 hours after delivery. Identification of hearing loss in the neonatal setting, in those hospitals, is a daily task. Otherwise, newborn babies are sent home without being screened.

It is prudent to screen all neonates in a particular setting so that many with hearing problems are not missed. When babies with hearing loss are not identified by a neonatal screening, they often are not identified until the school screening, when they are 5 or 6 years old. By that time, a hearing-impaired child may have suffered significant language and learning delay.

ASHA (1989) has published specific guidelines for identification of hearing loss in the neonatal setting, which recommend the use of a hearing high-risk register (Joint Committee, 1982) in all neonatal units and ABR screening for those neonates identified as high risk. In an analysis of the ASHA guidelines, Turner (1990) pointed out the need to determine what methods are efficient in the identification of neonatal hearing impairment. Further research may determine efficient methods for the identification of neonatal hearing impairment. Oto-acoustic emission (OAE) audiometry shows promise of providing a cost-efficient means for universal infant hearing screening. Once such methods are developed, neonatal hearing screening will become more widely available. Recently, the National Institute of Health (NIH) examined the need for universal infant screening and in a draft conference statement recommended universal infant hearing screening (NIH, 1993).

The purpose of identifying neonates with hearing problems is to make parents aware of their children's needs and to recommend treatment. Regular and persistent follow-up of each neonate identified as at risk for hearing loss is essential. Parents should also be made aware that annual hearing evaluations are necessary to identify progressive or acquired hearing loss in children who are at high risk for hearing loss but who passed the neonatal screening.

Noise Survey

Noise in the neonatal setting is of two types: ambient and electrical. **Electrical noise** may result from poor shielding of adjacent equipment or improper grounding, so that electrical activity from adjacent equipment produces interference during recording. As in any setting, the ambient noise level can be determined with the use of a SLM and an octave band analyzer. Electrical noise is an important consideration in the environment of the neonatal unit because most of the screening involves physiological recording of bioelectrical potentials. Most hospital equipment is shielded and properly grounded. However, do not take the possibility of electrical noise lightly. Always do preliminary runs without stimulation to detect patterns of electrical interference.

Education

The supervisor usually is responsible for educating facility personnel regarding the screening function. The supervisor may involve practicum students. Education in the neonatal setting involves five groups: hospital and unit administrators, unit staff, parents, obstetricians, and pediatricians. Regular contact with administrators is important. Telephone calls and notes alerting unit supervisors to previously scheduled visits to well baby and intensive care neonatal units for hearing screening may be effective in maintaining lines of communication. Quarterly reports on program progress are an effective tool for educating administration and keeping the program visible to administrators.

Regular inservices to the staff are important. Staff turnover in hospital neonatal units may be high. Unless care is taken to educate new staff as they arrive and refresh continuing staff concerning their roles and the program's goals, the neonatal identification program will be undermined rapidly. Education of staff is accomplished best in a scheduled staff meeting. In neonatal units, staff is divided into three shifts. As in nursing homes, the number of staff meetings may be reduced by meeting between two shifts.

The initial inservice for staff should take place a day or two before the screening takes place, so that staff have an opportunity for input and involvement. A day or two allows staff enough time to prepare for the screening without unduly interrupting previously scheduled activities. An inservice scheduled more than a day or two in advance of the initial screening may be too far removed from the screening to generate the level of staff interest and cooperation desired.

Parents should receive education about the program. There are several opportunities to present the program to the parents. Many first-time parents attend parenting classes offered by the hospital staff. Arrangements should be made for a representative of the neonatal hearing conservation team to present the program to the parents, to educate parents about hearing, auditory development, hearing loss and its effects, and management strategies for neonates. Interaction should be encouraged and parents' questions answered. Practicum students may participate in these parent education and counseling sessions. Clinical contact hours may be obtained for this activity and should be recorded as the student would hours for counseling parents of children participating in any other clinical service.

Some parents do not attend preparenting classes offered at the hospital. In such cases, it is important to spend a short time with the mother after she has given birth and before she and the baby are released. Time spent with each mother is limited by the number of personnel available, the comfort of the mother, and the number of mothers to be contacted. Therefore, the information presented must be simple, clear, and to the point. All mothers should receive a handout summarizing the program and their responsibility in it. In some facilities, nursing staff may be able and willing to perform this function and can be trained to do so through staff inservice. Parent education is an extremely important phase of the hearing conservation program.

A part of many hearing conservation programs in neonatal settings involves the use of a high-risk register. ASHA recommends the use of a 7-point high-risk register in all neonatal units (ASHA, 1989). Attending physicians or attending nurses should complete a checklist form high-risk register immediately following the birth of a child. Physicians may be provided the form in the mother's chart which is filled out and transferred to the neonate's chart. A short written explanation of the purpose of the high-risk register should be mailed to all physicians who have delivery privileges at the hospital. As new physicians come to practice at the hospital, a short written explanation of the program, including the high-risk register, should be included in their orientation materials.

Education of pediatricians is another important part of the neonatal hearing conservation program. The pediatrician also is capable of completing the high-risk register and will be able to complete forms not completed by the physician attending the delivery. The pediatrician is the health care specialist who will have the most regular contact with the child for the first years of life. He or she is in the most advantageous position to ensure periodic screening and follow-up audiologic diagnosis and treatment for children identified as at risk for hearing loss. A marketing campaign to educate and enlist the support of pediatricians is imperative. Mailings, guest presentations at county medical societies, and participation in grand rounds are all vehicles that can be used to educate and to gain the support of pediatricians.

Identification

Behavioral screening of neonates is impractical. Special equipment, like the crib-o-gram, has been developed for screening neonates. Immittance screening audiometry, ABR, and OAE audiometry are three physiological techniques available for screening neonates. The equipment for these tests is relatively expensive to purchase and to operate. Hospitals are reluctant to invest in expensive procedures without some method of recouping their costs.

Currently, few hospitals assign resources to neonatal hearing screening. Unless the equipment is made available through grant money, the audiology department in the hospital or the hearing conservation service contracted has to provide the necessary equipment.

Neonates are not moved to and from the screening area. The equipment and testing personnel are moved to the neonatal unit. The student participating in practicum that requires entrance into a neonatal unit must have current vaccinations and exercise precautions prescribed to protect the health of the newborns.

The student in this practicum setting needs to be familiar with electrophysiological test variables and techniques of electrically shielding test equipment from other electrical units. The student also must be knowledgeable regarding pediatric audiological concerns. These areas usually are covered in more advanced graduate course work. The first semester clinician is not likely to be involved in identification audiometry involving physiologic testing. Third or fourth semester graduate audiology practicum students are more likely to have the background to participate in neonatal identification audiometry.

An objective and noninvasive method of establishing cochlear function is OAE testing (Decker, 1992). Clinical OAE testing was introduced in North America from England in the early 1990s. This technique stimulates the ear with a complex sound and measures sound energy emitted from the cochlea in response to the sound. Used in conjunction with immittance and ABR screening, a rather complete picture of a neonate's ability to respond to sound may be obtained.

Immittance screening should include tympanometry, volume, and reflex measures to define middle ear function. A suggested ABR screening would use a 40 dB nHL, or less, click in each ear (Joint Committee on Infant Hearing, 1991).

A difficulty to be surmounted with any program to identify hearing impairment in neonates is how the cost is to be covered. This is an issue that must be resolved in the future.

In hospital neonatal units the day of the week and the time of day when screenings are conducted are less important than in other settings. The time needed to screen the hearing of neonates varies with their arousal state, the amount of screening to be done, and the skill of the tester. If the neonate is asleep and if the screening is limited to ABR at 40 dB nHL, the total screening time will be under 30 minutes. Total screening time includes locating the equipment, prepping the neonate, placing the electrodes, obtaining tracings for each ear, removing the electrodes, and recording the tracings.

Reporting

In the neonatal setting, as in other settings, reports serve as vehicles for public relations, marketing, and program review. The report should contain a description of the program, the vital statistics of the program, and examples of human interest associated with the program. Neonatal programs often distribute in-house reports on a quarterly basis. The fourth quarterly report can be written as an annual report, utilizing an attractive format for public relations. Copies may be sent to audiologists and physicians in the community. All reports should be mailed with a cover letter thanking each individual for his or her cooperation and encouraging support for continuation of the service.

Quarterly reporting can be accomplished by written report and by oral presentation before administrative meetings. During these contacts, the purpose of the program and the program components are reviewed for the administrators.

Follow-Up Services

The child identified as being at risk for hearing loss must be tested at regular intervals as he or she grows older. ASHA recommends that individuals identified as having hearing loss be referred to a clinical facility for diagnostic testing before 6 months of age. Some programs deliver many of the services needed in the hospital setting.

Neonatal hearing screening programs are instituted to identify children at risk for hearing impairment. The purpose of identifying children with hearing problems is to make parents aware of their needs and to encourage treatment. If the parent has been made aware of the child's problems, it is important to know if the child is being managed. A member of the neonatal hearing conservation team should maintain contact with families of children who have been identified as at risk for hearing loss.

Knowing what treatment is appropriate for the neonate at risk for hearing loss begins with diagnostic hearing testing, ideally before the child is 6 months old. The neonatal hearing conservation program should maintain contact with area audiologists, as well as physicians.

Program Evaluation

In addition to an evaluation of program efficiency related to stated program goals, a cost/income analysis is often required in neonatal screening programs. In today's hospital setting, unless a service generates income or reduces cost, it will not be offered for long. Income to the hospital from a neonatal hearing screening program may be indirect, resulting from increased referrals to the hospital's diagnostic audiology services, but it must be shown to be there in some form.

Cost savings to the hospital may result from replacing a more expensive screening technique with a less expensive one.

Like some hearing conservation programs in other settings, programs in the neonatal setting are continuous. Therefore, quarterly program reviews are more convenient than annual reviews alone.

9
The Workplace Setting

Hearing conservation in the workplace typically is found in industrial and military settings where employees are exposed to excessive noise. Hearing conservation programs in workplace environments are regulated under federal and state law. For private industries engaged in interstate commerce, the law is based on the Occupational Safety and Health Act (OSHAct) and the regulations published and enforced by the Occupational Safety and Health Administration (OSHA) (OSHA, 1983). For workplace environments that are considered to have special safety considerations, or are critical to the national defense, special regulations are established by their individual regulating bodies. For example, for the military, the regulatory agency is the Department of Defense; for mining, it is the Bureau of Mines; for transportation, the Department of Transportation; and so on. In most respects, many of these special regulations are similar to those applied to industry in general. However, students in practicum must become familiar with the regulations governing the group with which they plan to work. For example, it is not unusual for an audiology practicum student to have an opportunity to participate in practicum at a military facility.

In addition to workplace noise that is regulated because it is loud enough to endanger hearing, workplace noise may interfere with efficient task management or be annoying to workers. There are published guidelines dealing with such instances (Kryter, 1985).

169

Some university clinical training programs conduct pre-employment testing, auditory monitoring, and even limited education of employees for small local firms. However, university clinical training programs seldom are staffed to meet industry's needs for a hearing conservation program.

University clinics can provide students in practicum with excellent experience conducting hearing conservation programs in workplace settings by establishing off-campus placements. Off-campus placements that allow the student to obtain practicum contact hours must be staffed by an ASHA certified audiologist. However, some hearing conservation services are offered by industrial medicine groups that do not employ audiologists. These practices are inappropriate for students in practicum because they cannot earn clinical clock hours. Technicians hired by audiologists to provide testing services also are not qualified to supervise student practicum.

The goals of hearing conservation programs in the workplace are to educate workers about hazards to their hearing in the workplace, identify pre-employment hearing loss to reduce the employer's liability, and monitor workers' hearing. The main objective is to prevent hearing loss potentially caused by the workplace environment.

A large industry may have a sound-treated room and a pure-tone audiometer for testing. Some industries have mobile testing facilities and may even hire their own audiologists. A few industries contract with local clinical facilities to provide services. Some industries use a combination of service models to meet their needs. Other industries contract with hearing conservation services.

A first semester practicum student is seldom involved in workplace hearing conservation. Because workplace hearing conservation is required by law and has complex medico-legal implications, employers usually accept only more advanced clinicians, and the activities of these clinicians may be limited as well.

All employees exposed to the equivalent of 85 dBA of noise in an 8-hour day and all new employees are required by law to have their hearing tested annually. New employees should be tested to identify hearing loss existing prior to employment. Employers are not responsible for employee hearing loss documented prior to employment.

Noise Survey

There are two concerns related to noise in the workplace:

• Noise levels that endanger hearing
• Noise levels that interfere with tasks.

To determine which workers are exposed to greater than 85 dBA for an 8-hour day, a noise survey of the plant is required. A small machine tool business may have all operations in a single room. A larger manufacturing concern may have several rooms within several large buildings that include activities that may result in excessive noise. Regardless of whether the excessive noise is of the type that harms hearing or interferes with tasks, the noise survey is accomplished by a series of steps:

• Verification of floor plan
• SLM measurements
• Data summary
• Recommendations

The only way to verify the floor plan and the manufacturing processes by area is to walk through the plant. You should take required safety precautions. Wear a hard hat and safety glasses in areas where they are required. Most importantly, wear your hearing protection. If you do not, workers cannot be expected to take hearing protection against noise seriously.

While walking through the facility, sketch equipment location and room dimensions. Use your sketches and the plans to make an up-to-date floor plan that accurately reflects equipment location, worker location, and activity. Once you are familiar with the layout of the facility, you may be able to eliminate some areas as absent activity or isolated from noise. Areas that are suspect for excessive noise levels should be measured.

Overall noise levels must be obtained in dBA. Workers in any area in excess of 85 dBA for an 8-hour work day must be provided a hearing conservation program. However, any area in excess of 90 dBA for an 8-hour work day requires that noise controls be implemented.

If noise in workplace settings is considered to be annoying or to be interfering with tasks, it should be measured utilizing a SLM and an octave band analyzer. Kryter (1985) has given a description of levels of noise compatible with various activities.

In addition to dBA measurements, octave band measurements should be obtained. Octave band measurements may reveal the source of excessive noise and assist maintenance engineers in reducing noise.

After SLM measurements are completed, data must be assembled and reported in a clear and concise manner.

Education

Education in the work place most often is accomplished in two stages. When the initial site visit is made, a conference with management is completed to explain the purpose of the hearing conservation program and its components. Methods used to educate the workers are determined. A time is set for baseline and follow-up hearing testing. Testing facilities are located. Plans are made for efficient scheduling and movement of workers to and from the testing area.

Often, management perceives the purpose of hearing conservation programs as identification of hearing problems. Identified hearing problems may be viewed as financial liabilities. It is important for management to realize that workplace-induced hearing loss and not the identification of it is the financial liability. With effective hearing conservation programs, workers are less likely to initiate compensation claims for workplace-induced hearing loss. For management, the primary goal of the hearing conservation program is to reduce company liability for hearing loss and to lower workman's compensation insurance premiums.

Education of workers is accomplished best one-on-one at the end of the test when results are discussed. However, companies have different policies on reporting results to workers. This is an extremely sensitive area in some industries, and the student in practicum must be certain that she or he stays within program guidelines concerning reporting data to employees. Some industries schedule health and safety workshops for their employees. An advanced practicum student may have an opportunity to conduct such a session. Because this is educational material presented directly to workers whose hearing is at risk, many supervisors consider it is appropriate to grant clinical clock hours to students in practicum who conduct such a session. However, the student must have appropriate course work on the effects of noise on hearing, the effective use of hearing protection on and off the job, and worker and management responsibility under the law.

In addition to scheduled group health and safety meetings, many programs also educate the workers individually during the presentation of their results after testing. Students in practicum may count time spent educating workers about the hazards of noise exposure as clinical contact hours.

Identification

To test hearing effectively in the workplace, the student in practicum must have completed study that familiarizes the student with workplace hearing conservation. Some of this information is provided in introductory course work in audiology. However, more detailed information regarding hearing conservation in the workplace is usually contained in graduate courses.

For hearing tests to monitor hearing threshold levels adequately, the tests must be administered in an environment with ambient noise levels low enough to allow threshold testing at 25 dB HL, the medico-legal limit of normal hearing. Table 9-1 gives the ambient noise levels allowable in an industrial testing environment. Industry is not concerned with hearing below the legally defined upper limit of normal hearing, 25 dB HL. An area in which ambient noise levels exceed these values is unacceptable for testing. Legally, ambient noise levels in the test environment must be measured and a record kept of the measurements, the equipment used to make the measurements, the date and time the measurements were made, and who made them.

Testing in the workplace is conducted at specific frequencies, and thresholds are determined down to 25 dBA. Anyone with hearing levels better than 25 dBA is considered to have normal hearing. Thus, 25 dBA becomes a "low fence" for hearing testing in the workplace. The frequencies mandated by law include 500, 1000, 2000, 3000, 4000, and 6000 Hz in each ear. Baseline testing is to occur within 6 months of employment, or a year if provided by contracted mobile

TABLE 9-1. Maximum allowable ambient noise levels (in dB SPL for octave bands) for audiometric test rooms acceptable to the Occupational Safety and Health Administration.

	FREQUENCY IN HERTZ				
CONDITION	500	1000	2000	4000	8000
Under earphones	40	40	47	57	62

Source: From *Federal Register.* (p. 9781) by OSHA, 1983, March 8, Occupational noise exposure; Hearing conversation amendment; Final rule. 48(46).

services. Employees who have a standard threshold shift of 10 dB or greater require additional testing.

There are several effective ways to coordinate the movement of persons to and from the testing area. Cooperative supervisors will ensure an even flow of workers to be tested.

Sound-treated mobile facilities capable of testing several individuals automatically are available. In the workplace, where hearing testing programs are mandated by law, such equipment often is purchased or services that utilize such equipment are contracted. The practicum student needs to be familiar with automatic audiometers, testing procedures with groups, and the computer storage and retrieval of test data.

Certain time constraints should be recognized in scheduling testing at an industrial site. Days on which other programs such as pulmonary and respiratory testing are scheduled should be avoided when scheduling hearing testing. The first and last days of the week often have a higher number of absentees than the middle three days of the week.

Reporting

Two separate reporting formats are needed for management in the workplace setting. One reporting format is directed to management, presenting the results from the noise survey and including suggestions for controlling noise. This report should be updated whenever changes in equipment or schedules result in changes in the noise exposure environment. The second reporting format involves a series of reports on identification audiometry and follow-up services. These reports should be submitted to management after regularly scheduled testing.

After SLM measurements are completed, data must be assembled and reported in a clear and concise manner. Areas where measurements are taken must be clearly designated, and measurements must be stated and referenced properly. When the data are assembled and organized, they are summarized and included in a report.

The noise survey report to management includes an introduction, the data summary, and the recommendations. Workers for whom a hearing conservation program must be provided should be listed by name, shift, supervisor, and section. Noise levels that exceed an equivalent 90 dBA level for an 8-hour day must be listed, and the recommendation made that noise control measurements be implemented.

Reports on the results of testing should be simple. The names of those tested, those for whom baselines were established, those with significant threshold shifts to be retested within 3 months, and those to be tested annually should be listed. The noise survey report serves to inform management of the company's hearing conservation needs. The report on the results of testing stimulates program review and informs the management. These reports should be clear, concise, and to the point.

Initially, a report on the noise survey, including recommendations, should be completed and submitted to management within 2 weeks of testing. After the initial report, annual reports that summarize program activity for the year are a good idea.

Follow-up Services

Ideally, follow-up services for individual workers include referral for audiological or medical consultation for individuals with significant hearing losses or suspected but medically treatable conditions. Often, when workers are referred by the hearing conservation service, they expect management to pay for services not be covered under their health plan. As a result, management may prefer that workers receive little or no information at the time of testing and may assume the entire responsibility for follow-up services. The authors recommend that the person in charge of the hearing conservation program be directly responsible for referral and follow-up, if possible. Whatever the appropriate follow-up, it should take place in a timely fashion and in compliance with the requirements of the law (OSHA, 1983). The report of the hearing conservation program should be sent to management and a copy of the report should be kept on file at the agency providing the service.

Program Evaluation

The effectiveness of the hearing conservation program in the workplace setting may be evaluated by different methods. For example, assessing compliance with current state and federal regulations is one method of evaluating of the effectiveness of a program. Periodic reviews of regulations are needed to see whether the work setting continues to comply.

The Federal Register contains federal regulations pertaining to noise and hearing conservation. In states that have noise regulations, regulatory agencies often mail notices of forthcoming program changes. The person in charge of the hearing conservation program must analyze the program in light of the law and ensure compliance. When a program is in compliance, it is effective because compliance prevents citations and fines.

Another measure of the effectiveness of the program is management's support for the program and knowledge of its goals and objectives. If workers wear their ear protection in noise on and off the job, that, too, is a measure of the effectiveness of the educational component of the workplace hearing conservation program.

Yet another method of evaluation is to examine hearing testing results over time. Serial audiograms should show few cases where hearing gets worse. For workers with progressive noise-induced hearing loss, the program is not working. However, some workers may suffer progressive hearing loss from factors other than noise. Serial audiograms also should show few instances of improved hearing in later audiograms. Seldom would large groups of workers simultaneously suffer and recover from conductive hearing losses of the same extent. When hearing in large groups improves significantly from one test to the next, testing validity is questionable.

Regardless of the setting, hearing conservation programs must meet their goals effectively. Determining whether programs meet their goals requires systematic program evaluation. If you find yourself a part of a hearing conservation program without an evaluation component, you should initiate one to determine the value of the experience. Of course, professional tactfulness is called for. A properly designed practicum experience in hearing conservation will choose situations with established evaluative components or insist that they be developed.

In Part II, various hearing conservation programs were outlined, and the role of the student in practicum was discussed. In Part III, diagnostic strategies will be introduced and discussed.

Part III

Identification of Auditory Problems: A Strategy

I n Part II of the text, you were introduced to hearing conservation programs and strategies for the successful completion of practicum in hearing conservation. In Part III you will be introduced to a strategy for diagnostic and communicative needs assessment in audiology. In some programs students in speech-language pathology tend to be involved primarily with an audiometric battery used to identify hearing status in clients seen initially for service. This battery involves taking a case history, cursory otoscopic examination, immittance, pure-tone air- and bone-conduction testing with masking as required, and speech audiometry. The step-by-step procedures for the administration and interpretation of these tests are taught in a basic audiometry course and are readily accessible for review in a variety of audiology books.

In addition to an initial audiometric test battery, students majoring in audiology will be expected to gain experience in advanced diagnosis. These experience include conducting behavioral tests for differential diagnosis, electronystagmography (ENG), evoked response audiometry (ERA), otoacoustic emission (OAE) testing, central auditory processing (CAP) evaluation, hearing aid evaluation, and communicative needs assessment. In Part III, you will be introduced to strategies for conducting diagnostic testing and needs assessment. Step-by-step procedures for audiologic diagnostic and communicative needs assessment will not be presented because these procedures are thoroughly covered in academic course work and are available in several excellent textbooks. Instead, the discussion in the two chapters of Part III will concentrate on developing a philosophy toward, an approach to, diagnostics that will guide you throughout your practicum experiences and into your clinical practice.

Auditory problems fall into two general classes. In one class are problems with active physical pathology requiring medical or surgical treatment. In the other class are problems that are untreatable medically or surgically, but as effectively managed by other means, or require management beyond medicine and surgery. The student should know the difference, so that he or she can inform the clients accurately about their conditions and educate them on their treatment options.

Audiologists provide a valuable service to physicians and surgeons by identifying hearing problems and administering tests that differentiate between types of hearing disorders. Audiologic diagnosis aids in medical diagnosis and treatment of conditions causing hearing loss. Many otorhinolaryngologists either employ audiologists or rely on audiologists working in hospitals and private clinics. A recent ASHA survey (*Asha*, 1992a) indicated that 24% of audiologists listed their primary employment in offices of private physicians. Another 21% indicated that they were employed in hospital settings. In other words, in the early 1990s approximately 45% of audiologists worked in settings designed to provide physicians assistance with medical and surgical diagnosis and treatment. Many of these practices go beyond strictly physician support and provide a variety of other services. Although the student speech-language pathologist enrolled in audiology practicum is unlikely to be assigned to supervised experience in off-campus medical settings, the student audiologist has a high probability of experiencing practicum in such a setting.

Regardless of the presence or absence of active pathology, the person with hearing loss often experiences communication problems that medicine or surgery cannot remediate. Those with active pathology requiring medical or surgical treatment should be called back to the audiologist to manage the communication problems resulting from their hearing loss.

Audiologic testing can identify and influence medical and surgical treatment options. However, audiologic diagnosis involves more than providing data for differential medical and surgical diagnosis and treatment. **Audiologic diagnosis** has as its purpose identifying hearing problems, management options, and guiding audiologic management of hearing and hearing-related problems. **Audiologic management** is aimed at maximizing communication for individuals with hearing impairment. In Part III, we will describe a strategy to identify auditory problems. In Part IV, we will present nonmedical, nonsurgical treatment options for individuals with hearing problems.

10

Assessing Auditory Problems

A udiology clinic and, therefore, audiology clinical practicum, involves the appropriate diagnosis and management of hearing problems. It is a purpose of **diagnostic audiology** to differentiate among peripheral and retrocochlear hearing losses and central auditory processing problems, to classify peripheral hearing loss into types, and to obtain specific information to guide the implementation of appropriate management techniques. The most common type of hearing problem identified from audiologic testing is the peripheral hearing problem. Methods of assessing peripheral and retrocochlear hearing loss and central auditory problems are discussed in this chapter.

Types of Organic Peripheral Hearing Loss

Peripheral hearing loss typically is classified into four major categories:

- Conductive
- Sensory
- Neural
- Mixed

Conductive Hearing Loss

Conductive hearing loss occurs whenever normal sensorineural potential for hearing is better than the actual hearing. In the general population, conductive hearing problems comprise less than 20% of all hearing losses. In the audiology practice associated with an otolaryngology practice, the percentage of conductive hearing problems seen will be higher than in the general audiology practice. In the audiology practice located in a pediatric medical setting, the percentage of conductive hearing problems seen is significantly higher. Several diagnostic procedures are employed to identify conductive hearing problems.

General Diagnostic Procedures

Visual examination of the pinna and otoscopic examination of the ear canal and surface of the tympanic membrane may reveal obvious irregularities. Structural irregularities indicate the possibility of hearing loss, often conductive hearing loss. Audiologists diagnose conductive hearing loss by comparing air- and bone-conduction test results. If the bone-conduction results are within normal limits and the air-conduction results are significantly worse, a conductive hearing loss exists. With the advent of immittance testing, conductive hearing loss can be identified in situations where pure-tone air- and bone-conduction test results do not yield definitive results such as conditions where overmasking occurs.

Today, audiologists still obtain pure-tone bone-conduction measurements to diagnose hearing potential and to shed light on the locus of middle ear problems. However, with the advent of immittance measures into the general clinical setting in the early 1970s, diagnosis of conductive hearing problems originating in the middle ear gained in sensitivity and specificity. A student in practicum will be expected to be familiar with the equipment and procedures required to accomplish visual inspection of the external ear, the ear canal, and surface of the tympanic membrane, and to conduct pure-tone air- and bone-conduction testing with masking as needed. The student also should be familiar with the immittance battery.

Causes of Conductive Hearing Loss

Conductive hearing losses may be congenital or acquired and may result from a variety of causes. These causes include obstruction in the outer or middle ear and collapsing ear canals.

The factors that cause the blockage of the ear canal occur with differential frequency. Rare in occurrence is an atresia/aplasia that blocks the transmission of sound to the cochlea. Atresia/aplasia conditions may be congenital. Sometimes they are the result of mechanical injury. Somewhat less rare, but rare nonetheless, is swelling or edema of the ear canal due to injury or allergy that results in closure that blocks transmission of the sound to the cochlea. **Osteomas** are benign bony tumors of the ear canal. Infrequently, osteomas block transmission of the sound through the ear canal to the cochlea. Also rare in occurrence is a foreign object in the ear large enough to block sound from the cochlea. The most common cause of conductive hearing loss from obstruction of the ear canal is impacted cerumen. Impacted ear wax probably accounts for less than 10% of the conductive hearing problems seen in the general population.

Ear wax does not have to be impacted, or even excessive, to interfere with some clinical procedures. A clean ear canal is desirable for making real-ear measurements; insert-earphone testing; earmold impressions; and for caloric stimulation during ENG evaluation.

Ear wax is a special concern in three populations: individuals with Down syndrome, elderly persons, and hearing aid users. Ear wax may impact in the ear canal and cause conductive hearing loss. It may block surgically implanted ventilation tubes and cause reoccurrence of middle ear effusion. Ear wax also may impact in earmolds of hearing aids and prevent amplified sound from reaching the auditory system.

Ear wax impaction occurs more often in elderly persons than in younger persons. In a number of elderly males, the cilia in the cartilaginous portion of the ear canal grow profusely. When combined with ear wax, the cilia produce a tough barrier to sound. Individuals who are hearing aid users are even more susceptible to ear wax impaction. In the general clinical population, these individuals may represent a small percentage of the cases seen. However, in a VA clinic, where the population is predominately elderly males, a significantly higher percentage of these individuals will be seen.

Hearing aid users, by the act of removing and inserting earmolds and in-the-ear hearing aids, impact ear wax into the canal. The greater the production of ear wax, the more likely ear canal or earmold blockage will occur. Unless effectively managed, a small but significant proportion of hearing aid users may experience problems. In addition to blocking sound, ear wax may cause feedback problems for hearing aid users.

Conditions that cause conductive hearing loss originating in the middle ear also occur with differential frequency. In the general clinical practice of audiology, we rarely see individuals with glomis jugularis or disarticulation of the ossicular chain. Somewhat more frequently, but still somewhat rarely, we see ossicular fixation in the general practice of audiology. The majority of the conductive hearing problems originating in the middle ear encountered in general audiology practice are from middle ear effusion. When fluid fills the middle ear, significant conductive hearing loss may result.

The largest population presenting with middle ear problems is of preschool and early elementary school age. At any one time, 30% of this population may have various kinds of middle ear problems. They show significantly deviant middle ear pressure or effusion. They may have surgically inserted ventilation tubes. Many of them may be on antihistamines and antibiotics for upper respiratory congestion. Children with a history of middle ear disorders should be monitored for eustachian tube function. The student should be familiar with eustachian tube evaluation procedures utilizing immittance.

The student clinician should be aware that a measured conductive hearing loss may result from a collapsed ear canal. This condition occurs when air-conduction testing is administered using a circumaural earphone cushion. It does not occur when insert earphones are used to test hearing. The pressure of the circumaural cushion on the ear canal from in front of the tragus causes a flaccid canal to collapse, producing a mild-to-moderate conductive hearing loss.

Elderly females are more prone to have flaccid ear canals than others. Therefore, whenever a conductive hearing problem is encountered during the testing of an elderly female, a collapsing ear canal should be suspected. An air-bone-conduction gap results from pure-tone testing while immittance indicates a normal conductive mechanism. Visual examination of the shape of the ear canal often will reveal that the canal has lost its rounded appearance and appears to be a narrow vertical slit. By placing slight pressure in front of the tragus with a finger, the canal may be observed to collapse. If available, insert earphones should be used to test these individuals.

Sensory Hearing Loss

Sensory hearing loss occurs when there is interference with the action of the hair cells in the cochlea. Hair cell action may be mechanically impeded or the hair cells may be damaged or destroyed. In the general clinical population, sensory hearing problems comprise the largest percentage of all hearing loss. In the audiology practice associated with an otolaryngological practice, sensory hearing losses will be the predominant type of hearing loss. However, as mentioned earlier, in the otolaryngological practice, more medically treatable conductive hearing problems are seen, and as a result, sensory hearing losses will not appear to dominate the caseload, as they do in the non-medical-based practice. In an audiology practice located in a pediatric medical setting, the percentage of sensory hearing problems is significantly lower than that of conductive hearing problems. In many hearing-aid-dispensing audiology practices, the percentage of clients with sensory hearing loss may approach 100%.

Often, in acquired sensory hearing loss, both the inner and outer hair cells are affected. However, some acquired conditions affect the inner and outer hair cells differentially. Nontramatic noise-induced hearing loss tends to affect outer hairs cell to a greater degree than inner hair cells. There are also some congenital conditions that affect outer or inner hair cells to a greater degree. The functions of the two types of hair cells differ, and their functions are well-enough understood to differentially diagnose the locus of sensory hearing loss as being inner, outer, or more global hair cell damage.

Outer Hair Cells

The three rows of outer hair cells in the human cochlea must be present for pure-tone threshold responses and otoacoustic emissions to occur. They appear to be involved in transforming relatively gross frequency and intensity information for signals below approximately 50 dB HL from mechanical to electrical information. Outer hair cells are involved when threshold sensitivity is reduced and when otoacoustic emissions are reduced or absent.

Inner Hair Cells

When the signal levels reach about 50 dB HL, inner hair cells begin to fire. The single row of inner hair cells is much more richly innervated than the outer rows of hair cells. Inner hair cell integrity is required for normal acoustic reflexes and for fine discrimination of intensity and frequency. The High Level Short Increment Sensitivity Index (HLSISI) is a test that requires discrimination of 1 dB increments of intensity superimposed on a carrier tone above 70 dB HL. Inability to identify 1 dB increments when the carrier tone is above 70 dB, an abnormal HLSISI, indicates decreased inner hair cell integrity or interference with information transmitted from the inner hair cells.

Currently, it is thought that, even if inner hair cells are absent, otoacoustic emissions may still exist at normal intensity levels. Theoretically, these cells could be absent in the presence of normal pure-tone threshold measurements. Amplification works better for sensory hearing loss when inner hair cells are less involved than outer hair cells. Speech discrimination improves when the amplified signal stimulates the more normal inner hair cells which are more capable than outer hair cells of finer intensity and frequency discrimination. Amplification introduced to compensate for hearing loss when there is significant loss of inner hair cells may not produce expected clarity, as measured by speech discrimination tests. Several diagnostic procedures that help to identify sensory hearing problems may be used to differentiate between conditions in which primarily inner hair cells are affected from those in which outer hair cells are affected.

General Diagnostic Procedures

As late as the early 1990s, audiologists and otolaryngologists preferred to group sensory and neural hearing loss into the category *sensorineural*. As a result of advances in understanding of auditory anatomy and physiology and advances in test equipment and procedures, audiologists are now capable of differentiating between sensory and neural sites of lesion.

Until the early 1970s and the advent of immittance testing, audiologists measured hearing by air- and bone-conduction and compared the results. If the bone-conduction results were abnormal and equal to air-conduction results, there was a sensorineural hearing loss. Today, audiologists still obtain pure-tone air- and bone-conduction measurements and infer sensorineural hearing loss from them. However, with immittance measures, audiologists can identify not only conductive hearing loss but also neural involvement through absent or decaying reflexes. Indirectly, normal reflexes without decay indicate sensory hearing loss. Moreover, purely outer hair cell sensory hearing loss of less than 50-60 dB HL should allow acoustic reflexes within normal ranges. The lack of reflex decay and a normal HLSISI test further rule out both neural and inner hair cell involvement.

In the mid-to-late 1970s, ABR was introduced clinically. Diagnostic procedures were developed whereby the possibility of neural involvement could be eliminated from purely sensory hearing losses. ABR provided yet another indirect indication of sensory hearing loss.

Then, in the early 1990s, otoacoustic emission measurement was introduced as an objective method of examining the integrity of the outer hair cells. With this measurement, audiologists could differentiate directly between inner and outer hair cell integrity within the category of sensory hearing loss.

As in a case of the collapsed canal in peripheral hearing loss, testing artifacts may indicate a sensory hearing loss when there is not one. When the distance between the eardrum and the diaphragm of the earphone is equal to 1/2 the wavelength of the tone presented, the reflected wave approaches 180° out of phase with the original wave and partial cancellation of the original tone results. The results suggest that the individual being tested has a high-frequency hearing loss at 6000 or 8000 Hertz (Hz). Why 6000 or 8000 Hz? Because those are the tones with the shortest wavelengths. The wavelength of a 4000 Hz tone is approximately 8.58 centimeters (cm). One half of 8.58 cm is 4.29 cm, which would be the length required for an ear canal to cause cancellation of a 4000 Hz tone. The distance between the eardrum and the diaphragm of the earphone in a very long ear canal may not approach 4.29 cm. The wavelength of an 8000 Hz tone is approximately 4.29 cm. In this case, the distance between the eardrum and the diaphragm of the earphone in an ear canal may approach 2.15 cm and result in cancellation of an 8000 Hz tone.

Whenever a sensory hearing problem is encountered at 6000 or 8000 Hz, a partial standing wave should be suspected. A partial standing wave may be broken up by having the client hold the earphone slightly away from the ear, thus creating a cavity open at one end and changing resonance from 1/2 to 1/4 of the wavelength. If the measured loss was from a partial standing wave, retesting of 8000 Hz with the earphone held away from the ear will result in better hearing. Use of insert earphones shortens the distance between the diaphragm of the earphone and the eardrum significantly, so that standing waves are not a problem when insert earphones are used routinely in testing.

As a beginning student in practicum, you will be expected to be familiar with the pure-tone and immittance equipment and procedures required to identify sensorineural hearing loss and to differentiate between sensory and neural hearing losses. Beyond the first semester of audiology practicum, the audiology student also may be required to be familiar with the equipment and procedures necessary to accomplish measurement of otoacoustic emissions and the auditory brainstem response. Some training programs rely on off-campus practicum facilities to train more advanced practicum students in the measurement of otoacoustic emissions and auditory brainstem response.

Causes of Sensory Hearing Loss

Sensory hearing loss may be congenital or acquired. **Congenital sensory hearing loss** may be genetic or acquired in utero. Cases of hearing loss resulting from genetic conditions are relatively rare. Cases of hearing loss resulting from conditions acquired in utero are increasing.

Increasing numbers of babies are being born with fetal alcohol syndrome, drug addiction, and low birth weights. These conditions put them at risk for sensory hearing loss. Increasing percentages of sensory hearing loss due to these causes are expected to be seen in the future, particularly in the pediatric audiology practice.

Acquired sensory hearing losses result from a variety of causes. They may result from mechanical injury, ototoxins, viral and bacterial infections, metabolic and vascular disorders, noise exposure, and the normal aging process.

In the general audiology practice, a sensory hearing loss resulting from mechanical injury is rarely seen. However, in some VA hospital settings and some specialized rehabilitation hospitals, a large percentage of hearing loss cases seen may be the result of mechanical injury. Somewhat less rarely in the general audiology practice, but rarely nonetheless, sensory hearing loss resulting from ototoxic influences may be seen. In burn hospitals and other critical care hospitals where life saving drugs with ototoxic side effects are administered, audiologists may spend the majority of their clinical time tracking ototoxic effects. Ototoxic effects are related to renal functioning. The weaker the kidneys, the longer the toxins remain in the system and, consequently, the greater the potential damage to hearing.

Viral infections may produce sensory hearing loss. Sometimes the unilateral, sudden, and complete hearing losses caused by viral infections are difficult to distinguish from sensory losses resulting from vascular accidents. With the expected increases in individuals who test positive for HIV, hearing loss related to viral and bacterial infections may increase dramatically over the next few years.

Vascular accidents produce sensory hearing loss by limiting cochlear blood supply. Vascular accidents and viral infections account for few of the sensory hearing losses seen in the general audiology practice. The most common causes of sensory hearing loss are noise exposure and the normal aging process. These two causes account for a majority of the sensory hearing losses seen in audiology clinics. Most individuals with sensory hearing loss related to noise exposure and the normal aging process have greater loss of outer hair cell function than inner hair cell function.

Peripheral Neural Hearing Loss

Peripheral neural hearing loss results from involvement of the auditory branch of the VIIIth cranial nerve. Neural hearing loss occurs when the transmission of the action potential of the auditory nerve fibers is interfered with. Conditions that slow, impede, or prevent transmission may interfere with the action potential of the nerve fiber. Auditory nerve cells may be damaged or destroyed and, therefore, unable to generate action potentials. Auditory nerve cells also may be subjected to pressure which can significantly slow conduction time of the action potentials to the brainstem. In addition, the nerve cells may not repolarize when blood supply is reduced and, therefore, be unable to sustain a response to a continuous signal. The cells may be intact but demyelinated, and, therefore, discharge at a significantly slower rate than normal.

General Diagnostic Procedures

Procedures that differentiate between sensory and neural hearing loss have evolved over the years. A differential battery of tests is called for under either of two conditions:

- Neural pathology is suspected because of a unilateral sensorineural hearing loss, poorer than expected speech discrimination scores, and reported neurological signs.
- There is no measurable hearing, and active pathology is not a concern.

When active neural pathology is suspected, the first concern is to identify the cause so that appropriate medical or surgical treatment can be applied. When there is no measurable hearing and active pathology is not a concern, neural stimulability is of interest in determining the individual's candidacy for a cochlear implant.

The beginning student in practicum must be aware of the conditions that indicate possible neurological involvement and referral for a differential audiologic test battery. First semester practicum students are seldom expected to administer and interpret advanced reflex studies, ABR, and other advanced differential diagnostic tests. More advanced practicum students, however, are expected to be familiar with the equipment and procedures necessary to accomplish a differential diagnosis.

The first tests thought to differentiate between neural versus sensory hearing loss were designed to identify individuals with active neural pathology. Clients so identified were referred for medical and surgical evaluation. For the most part, these tests lacked good sensitivity and are seldom used today. They have given way to more definitive measures.

Early differential tests included the Low Level Short Increment Sensitivity Index (LLSISI) administered at threshold plus 20 dB HL, Alternate Binaural Loudness Balance (ABLB) and Monaural Loudness Balance tests (MLB), Bekesy audiometry, and tone decay testing. The differential sensitivity of a battery incorporating these tests was only fair. Surgeons routinely relied on radiographic studies to identify tumors they could treat surgically.

With the immittance test battery came reflex and reflex decay testing which was found to have good differential sensitivity in discriminating between sensory and neural causes of hearing loss. With the incorporation of ABR into the routine of the general audiology practice, a most sensitive measure of neural integrity became available. The early differential tests are seldom used by the modern audiologist. Today, the audiologist either has the equipment to do more definitive testing or refers clients to nearby facilities that do.

The modern surgeon places greater confidence in the results of differential audiological assessment battery. When he or she receives a referral with neurological signs from an audiologist on the basis of immittance and ABR testing, he or she uses magnetic resonance imaging (MRI) to locate and measure the tumor, determine its operatibility, and guide the surgical treatment approach.

Several other diagnostic procedures are used in the evaluation and surgical treatment of neural pathology. Procedures often requested in the medical setting and administered by audiologists include electronystagmography (ENG) and posturography, transdermal stimulation and evaluation, and intraoperative monitoring.

Recall from your courses in anatomy and physiology that the internal auditory meatus in the temporal cephalic area provides a channel from the inner ear to the brainstem that is occupied by the vestibular as well as the auditory branch of the VIIIth cranial nerve. Additionally, the internal auditory meatus provides a channel to the more distal structures of the head for the facial nerve, cranial nerve VII, and the internal auditory artery. Therefore, a space-occupying lesion in the area of the internal auditory meatus may affect the vestibular system, innervation to the facial muscles, and blood supply to the inner ear.

The ENG battery provides a definitive assessment of dizziness problems. It assesses vestibular, postural, occulomotor, and central nervous system integrity. When interpreted in light of audiometric and other electrophysiologic measurements, the results of the ENG battery provide information concerning the locus of neuronal problems, whether they are peripheral vestibular, peripheral occulomotor, postural, or central. ENG is a fairly common diagnostic tool in most medical settings. The advanced student in practicum in a medical setting may be expected to know how to administer and interpret the basic ENG battery. Some training programs rely on off-campus practices in medical settings to provide practical training for ENG.

A relatively recent development for the evaluation of the client with dizziness is posturography. **Posturography** evaluates each sensory system that contributes to maintaining balance, separately and in combination, and central nervous system integration of the information from the sensory systems. Sensory systems that contribute to maintaining balance are the vestibular system, the occulomotor system, and the postural system. Posturography does a more thorough job of examining the dynamics of balance and posture than an ENG battery alone. Medical centers that see large numbers of clients with dizziness may employ this diagnostic tool. Learning to conduct posturography and to interpret the results is not difficult. Few university training programs outside medical settings currently have posturography units or are able to justify the purchase of a unit.

In addition to the assessment of the client with dizziness, the audiologist may administer electrically evoked responses to evaluate a variety of systems. Transtympanic stimulation of the promotory to assess auditory nerve function is discussed later in conjunction with evaluation to determine candidacy for cochlear implant. Facial nerve evaluation involves the stimulation and measurement of facial nerve integrity with clients experiencing facial numbness, paralysis, or both. Somatosensory evaluation uses electrical stimulation to evaluate large muscle responses. For the student trained in ABR, these electrophysiologic techniques are not difficult to learn. Like posturography, the student is most likely to come into contact with these procedures in the large otolaryngology practice. Audiology training programs seldom prepare students by more than an academic introduction in these areas prior to off-campus placement.

Another area associated with audiology in medical settings is **intraoperative monitoring**, which most often consists of monitoring the facial or auditory nerve responses during surgery. An audiologist monitoring neural responses can see changes in the nerves in response to surgical manipulation and inform the surgeon of the effects of such manipulations as they happen. This feedback allows the surgeon to alter procedures and to avoid unnecessary damage to the facial nerve or auditory system. At present, intraoperative monitoring is limited to a few very sophisticated medical facilities around the world. The practicum student interested in experience in this specialized area must seek practicum placement in one of these facilities.

In the recent past, audiology initiated diagnostic procedures for individuals who have no useful or measurable hearing to determine their **candidacy for cochlear implant.** When an active pathology affecting the health and well-being of the candidate has been ruled out or successfully treated, the main concern is to bypass the nonfunctional cochlea and to provide direct electrical stimulation to the intact VIIIth cranial nerve.

Development of implantable multipolar electrodes allows sound frequency information to be represented by place of stimulation and intensity information to be represented by rate of stimulation and the number of fibers stimulated. Thus, the encoding of sound waves as electrical events provides the VIIIth nerve with information in a manner similar to a functioning cochlea. Many recipients of multipolar cochlear implants are able to communicate in near-normal aural and oral fashion. Of course, postsurgical implantation requires fine tuning the speech processor of the cochlear implant used, discrimination training for the user, and other long-term management.

The diagnostic protocols used to determine candidacy for cochlear implants are different for children and adults. When time permits, children are fitted with hearing aids, and possibly tactile devices, to determine whether they can benefit from these devices in lieu of cochlear implants. The results of these trials are added to psychological, medical, and other considerations in determining candidacy for a cochlear implant.

With adults, a diagnostic procedure that is difficult to justify with children may be used. That procedure is transtympanic electrical stimulation of the promotory in the middle ear. The procedure is designed to measure VIIIth nerve response to electrical stimulation. It requires inserting a needle electrode through the tympanic membrane and the introduction of electrical stimulation. Responses may be measured by ABR and the client may report a sensation which is an additional indicator of VIIIth nerve response. Audiologists in medical settings often are involved in the stimulation of the promotory and measurement of the VIIIth nerve response. The advanced practicum student may be trained to participate with the surgeon in transtympanic electrical stimulation of the promotory.

Causes of Neural Hearing Loss

Several conditions can produce VIIIth nerve problems. However, in the general population of individuals with hearing loss, those with VIIIth nerve loss are relatively rare. Most profound hearing losses are sensory, not neural. A greater proportion of VIIIth nerve disorders will be encountered in audiology associated with otolaryngological or neurological practices.

The majority of VIIIth nerve disorders result from two conditions: tumors and demyelinating diseases such as multiple sclerosis. The VIIIth nerve tumor is the most common cranial tumor. Most are benign and many do not grow. Some exist in the internal auditory canal exerting less pressure on the auditory nerve and more on the internal auditory artery which supplies nutrients to the inner ear. Some relatively small tumors that produce a great deal of compression to the auditory nerve may be present. Because of these and other factors, amount of hearing loss and tumor size are only generally related.

Demyelinating diseases cause the myelinated VIIIth nerve fibers to become demyelinated. **Myelin** is the white fatty substance found on some nerve fibers. Myelin serves two functions:

- Insulation of fibers from one another
- Facilitation of conduction time.

When myelin is absent, there is a spread of activity across fibers and a slowing of conduction time. The slowing of conduction time is readily measured with ABR audiometry.

Mixed Hearing Loss

Mixed hearing loss occurs when the bone-conduction test results are abnormal but significantly better than the air-conduction results.

In the general population, mixed hearing losses are less prevalent than conductive hearing losses. In an audiology service associated with an otolaryngological practice, the percentage of mixed hearing losses seen will be higher than in the general audiology practice. In an audiology practice located in a pediatric medical setting, the percentage of mixed hearing loss may be higher than in a general practice but still not a significant portion of the total caseload.

General Diagnostic Procedures

The diagnostic procedures employed to identify mixed hearing losses are the same as those used to identify conductive and sensorineural hearing losses. To specify the amount of the conductive versus sensorineural components of the loss great care must be taken to mask appropriately.

Causes of Mixed Hearing Loss

Mixed hearing losses may result from a single condition that affects the conductive and the sensorineural mechanism or from unrelated conditions such as otosclerosis and noise-induced hearing loss. Some of these conditions were discussed in the previous sections dealing with conductive, sensory, and neural hearing losses.

Be thorough in your testing. Understand and use masking appropriately. Incorrect first impressions with mixed hearing losses at best delay appropriate treatment. At worst, they may result in inappropriate or even harmful treatment. For example, surgery designed to improve the conductive component of a supposed mixed hearing loss may be performed on an ear that, with proper masking, would have been identified as the having sensorineural loss.

Nonorganic Peripheral Hearing Loss

Nonorganic hearing loss is identified when the client reports a greater hearing loss than he or she actually has. Nonorganic hearing loss should be suspected when some test results are inconsistent with other test results in the battery, when the client is able to answer questions at quiet conversational levels without visual cues, and when the client stands to gain financially by having a hearing loss. There are several reasons for persons showing a greater hearing loss than they actually have. Some of the causes of nonorganic peripheral hearing loss are discussed in more detail later. Traditionally, individuals with non-organic peripheral hearing loss are subdivided into two groups:

- those who malinger
- those who have psychogenic problems.

Malingering implies that the individual is attempting to produce results that indicate hearing loss when none exists or a greater hearing loss than what exists. Such a person is fully aware of what he or she is doing. Malingering behavior often involves financial gain. Documented hearing loss may result in disability payments or damage settlements from accidents. An individual with such a hearing loss also may gain other, less tangible, benefits such as attention.

Psychogenic problems imply that an individual who produces results suggesting hearing loss does so without being aware of it. Such persons are not intentionally deceiving anyone. Some experts believe that psychogenic hearing loss may result from an individual's inability to cope with difficult life situations.

Persons with nonorganic hearing loss represent a small percentage of those assessed in a general audiometric practice, although some practices see a larger number of such cases. For example, an audiologic practice under contract to a state department of disability will see a proportionately higher percentage of malingerers than will a general audiology practice.

In the past, the majority of maligerers were adult males. This was because, until recently, adult females did not enlist in significant numbers into military service and few adult females were the primary family wage earners. After the Vietnam War, the number of active service personnel presenting with nonorganic hearing loss decreased sharply, but the number of former military personnel and refugees from Southeast Asia presenting with the same type of hearing loss when applying for VA or other benefits increased. During post-war and peace-time, the majority of nonorganic hearing losses are related to adult males' claims to job-related disability benefits.

When a nonorganic hearing loss is suspected, the clinician must resist urges to judge the client's motives. It is imperative to maintain objectivity and courtesy. At the same time, confronting the individual with inconsistent results may be appropriate. Often, critical medico-legal considerations accompany nonorganic hearing loss. At the first suspicion of nonorganic peripheral hearing loss, students in practicum are advised to inform their supervisors immediately, and to seek guidance.

General Diagnostic Procedures

If a client is referred by an attorney, or the stated reason for hearing loss on the case history form is accident- or work-related, the possiblity of nonorganic peripheral hearing loss is greater. The possibility of legal action also is great.

Informal Procedures

In addition to the standard audiometric battery, the audiologist will initiate other procedures. For example, after the initial interview in which rapport is established with the client, the clinician is careful to find opportunities to converse with the client at low intensity levels without visual contact by the client. A sure sign of nonorganic hearing loss is an ability to answer questions at levels below the client's admitted threshold and without visual contact.

Formal Procedures

Some audiologists anticipate that their results may be used as evidence in legal proceedings and take the precaution of performing a formal sound level calibration check on the equipment to be used immediately prior to and following the evaluation. Most audiologists interrupt testing to reinstruct the client regularly. Many audiologists confront the client with inconsistent results, reinstruct, and retest. If the validity of the audiometric results is still in question, special tests may be employed to identify nonorganic hearing loss.

With malingerers, unilateral nonorganic hearing loss is more common than bilateral nonorganic hearing loss because it allows the client to respond normally to conversation. The pure-tone or speech Stenger test may be used with suspected unilateral nonorganic hearing loss. This test is based on the principle that the individual to whom a signal is presented in both ears will hear the signal only in the ear where it is louder. If the signal in the ear with hearing loss is below the client's admitted threshold and the signal in the normal ear is slightly above threshold, the client will stop responding to the signal when the hearing loss is nonorganic. Of the early tests used to identify nonorganic hearing loss, only the Stenger has been retained.

With the advent of immittance testing, ABR, and otoacoustic emissions, objective measures of thresholds are possible in uncooperative clients. Because the clients with nonorganic hearing losses are considered uncooperative, the use of these procedures with them is justified. ABR and otoacoustic emissions cannot be fooled. If there is hearing, these two electrophysiological measures will indicate it. Thresholds can be estimated within 10 dB HL with ABR.

Immittance procedures may be used to identify thresholds that are normal versus mild-to-moderate or severe. First, when reflexes occur within normal limits (70-90 dB HL), sensory hearing loss can be no worse than 50-60 dB HL. Second, the amount and slope of an individual's hearing can be predicted by Differential Loudness Summation procedures. In these procedures, reflexes to pure tones are compared with reflexes to noise. The only way that an individual with nonorganic hearing loss can interfere with the measurement of acoustic reflexes is to refuse to sit still, clench and unclench his or her jaw, or behave in other ways to disrupt testing. However, refusal to cooperate in the testing procedure does not advance the client's case.

Causes of Nonorganic Hearing Loss

As mentioned earlier, nonorganic hearing loss results from malingering or psychogenic causes. Beyond that classification, causes are related to individual circumstances.

The student in practicum should examine each case of suspected nonorganic hearing loss carefully and ask the following questions.

- What referral information suggests nonorganic hearing loss?
- What inconsistent behavior on the part of the client suggests nonorganic hearing loss?
- What tests were chosen and why? What testing would be appropriate if these cases were seen in the completely equipped clinic?
- How is nonorganic hearing loss reported?
- What probable reasons did each case have for presenting with nonorganic hearing loss?

The following six cases illustrate varied individual circumstances, case histories, and assessment information that strongly suggested no hearing loss was present.

Case 1

A man in his late 20s was accompanied by his wife to the evaluation. His appointment had been scheduled through a local attorney. His wife answered the questions directed to him and insisted on accompanying him into the testing area. She was instructed to wait in the control booth while the client was instructed and prepared for testing. The audiologist stood between the wife on the other side of the viewing window and the client. The client was seated so that he faced opposite the viewing window; the audiologist was located behind the client. The audiologist placed the earphones on the client and asked several casual questions at a low level. The client responded appropriately to each without hesitation. The audiologist then left the client in the examination room and commenced testing. The wife was present during the testing.

Pure-tone results indicated moderate-to-severe sensorineural hearing loss. Pulsed tones were presented. Response consistency was fair. Speech reception thresholds indicated mild hearing loss. Immittance testing revealed no conductive hearing problems and reflexes within the normal range. Differential Loudness Summation revealed responses within normal limits. ABR and otoacoustic emission testing were not available. The testing was interrupted several times, and the client was reinstructed.

Results were reported to the client with his wife present. The audiologist explained that the results were inconsistent and encouraged the client to return for additional testing to determine the exact extent of any hearing loss he might have. The wife declined further testing for the client and instead described tinnitus as an additional problem experienced by her husband. The client sat passively through the process, but signed a release form for the results to be sent to his attorney. The wife asked what the report to the attorney was going to say. She was told that the report would say that the results of the testing were inconsistent. She asked to rescind the permission for the release of the information to their attorney. She was given the release form.

Several days later, the client's attorney telephoned requesting a copy of the report. He was considering representing this client in a claim against his employer for negligence that the client said had resulted in hearing loss. The attorney was told that a release form signed by the client and payment for services were required before a report could be sent. The attorney sent a check for the services and a signed release of information to the audiologist. A report, summarizing the inconsistencies and concluding that the hearing loss reported was nonorganic was sent to the attorney.

Subsequent to receiving the report, the attorney telephoned the audiologist and discussed the case. His question was, "Is this guy lying about his hearing loss?" The audiologist wisely answered that the hearing loss reported by the client did not represent how the client actually heard. Even though this case appears to be a cut-and-dried example of malingering, the client's motives are not open to judgment by the audiologist.

Case 2

She was 17 years old and the youngest of 10 children of a prominent local family. She was quiet and did not smile. She would not look the examiner in the eye. Her answers were slow and short. Her father, a member of the clinic's Board of Directors, was concerned with her grades which were average. He felt that she might have a hearing loss and scheduled her to be tested.

Preliminary pure-tone and speech test results revealed a bilateral mixed hearing loss. Immittance indicated normal middle ear function and reflex thresholds within normal limits. The audiologist retested pure-tone air-conduction thresholds and obtained results better by 15 dB. The client was rescheduled for the next week.

Results from pure-tone retesting were worse than original results by more than 25 dB. Differential Loudness Summation, ABR, and oto-acoustic emission testing were not available. The audiologist confronted the client with the results of the testing.

The confrontation was conducted in an understanding, kind manner. It began by the audiologist asking the client how she liked school, to which she replied that her brothers and sisters had done so much better in school than she. When asked to tell the audiologist about her siblings, the client described highly intelligent, motivated, and successful persons. When asked what her special interests were, she replied that she was good at nothing. She implied that she was disappointing to her parents.

When told that her responses to the hearing tests were inconsistent, she explained that at some times she appeared to hear worse than at other times. The audiologist expressed understanding that hearing was more difficult at some times than others, but reassured her that there was nothing wrong with her ears. At that point the client began to cry and stated, "I am so tired of not being good enough. I wish I were dead!"

With the client's permission, the parents were telephoned and asked to come into the clinic. Both rearranged their schedules and came in. The audiologist met with the parents, explained the situation, and secured their agreement that family counseling was important. A referral was made and an appointment set prior to conducting a closing interview with the client and her parents together.

In this case, whether the nonorganic hearing loss is psychogenic or the result of malingering is not important. It is possible the client intentionally reported hearing loss as a safe way to call for help. It was not as important to classify this hearing loss as psychogenic or malingering as it was to refer the client and her family for appropriate services.

Case 3

The child was a small second grader from a rural elementary school. He was tested after he had failed the school hearing screening and was referred by the school nurse. The nurse transported him to the clinic. His pure-tone test results revealed a 50 dB HL sensorineural hearing loss. His speech reception threshold was 40 dB HL. He was rescheduled for testing.

A different examiner saw the boy on his second visit. Test results revealed a 30 dB HL sensorineural hearing loss. The child was scheduled for a third visit and discovered by a third examiner to have hearing within normal limits.

It is interesting to note that the first examiner used a 50 dB HL model tone at which to begin testing. The second examiner used a 30 dB HL model tone at which to begin testing; whereas the third examiner used no model tone but began testing by ascending from -10 dB HL until a response was obtained. The youngster was confronted with his inconsistent responses and asked if he was having any problems. The following circumstances then came to light.

The client lived in a house trailer with his mother and younger sister in a remote area. Two months earlier, the father had been arrested for posession of drugs and was incarcerated. The family was in desperate circumstances with no utilities or food. There was no other family and no friends were aware of their plight. The mother was not aware of available social services.

The case was brought to the attention of the local county social worker who contacted his counterpart in the adjacent county in which the family resided. Services were procured for the family. In this case, a little boy's nonorganic hearing loss was a cry for help. This case illustrates an important point about the highly individual nature of the causes for presenting with nonorganic hearing loss. The audiologist should go beyond the obvious.

Case 4

He was an old man, a poor lay preacher of a small rural church. Recently, he had needed glasses and discovered that the state would purchase them for him. He had been scheduled at his request for a hearing test.

Initial test results were inconsistent. When confronted with the inconsistency and reinstructed, he confessed through tears to deliberately producing results worse than his actual hearing. When asked why, he stated that he thought it was such a wonderful thing when the state bought him glasses that he would just get a hearing aid, too. He expressed shame at his behavior and was very concerned that he was going to be sent to prison.

The audiologist reassured the client that his actions resulted more from confusion than they did from intent to do wrong. The audiologist composed the report in the man's presence, simply stating that his hearing was normal and no further services were required at this time. Furthermore, the audiologist assured the client that he was welcome to return for hearing re-evaluation as needed and that this session in no way would affect his eligibility for future services. This unusual case illustrates the importance of compassion and respect in dealing with individuals.

Case 5

A man and his wife scheduled simultaneous appointments. She was deaf with no measurable hearing. He wore powerful binaural body aids which he had purchased from a hearing aid dealer. He was proficient in both manual and oral communication.

Initial test results for the husband were inconsistent. When confronted with the inconsistency, the client retested with normal hearing. He explained that he loved his wife very much, but that, as a hearing person, he would not be accepted as readily by the deaf community. The audiologist questioned the client's assumptions about his acceptance into the deaf community, but agreed to keep his audiometric results confidential. The client was advised to wear the hearing aids turned off or without batteries, if he felt that he must wear them. This case further demonstrates the highly individual nature of the reasons persons present with nonorganic hearing loss.

Case 6

She was 11 years old and wore glasses. Her father, a local physician, brought her to the clinic for an annual hearing evaluation. She wore binaural body hearing aids prescribed for a severe sensorineural hearing loss a year before by clinic in another state where her father had been in medical school. She was an only child whose mother had died shortly before her father began medical school. Testing revealed hearing within normal limits after initial inconsistent test results.

In the conference room, the father was informed of the test results and counseled that he and his daughter were in need of professional counseling. He appeared calm and agreed to schedule family counseling with his daughter. Later, in the waiting room, in front of the receptionist and several other clients, he angrily confronted the child and tore the hearing aids from her. They left together with the father dragging the crying child behind him.

About a month after the hearing test, the child was killed because she stepped off a curb in front of a car. In the newspaper article about her death, the father reported taking the child's glasses from her after he discovered that "she had been faking visual problems." Were this child's nonorganic sensory problems psychogenic? Was her tragic accident due to an intense and unhappy emotional state?

This sad case illustrates two important points:

- Nonorganic hearing loss is often symptomatic of other problems.
- It is important to follow up on recommendations.

Because of the highly idiosyncratic reasons behind nonorganic hearing loss, the preceding cases were presented. They illustrate several important points to be remembered in dealing with individuals who present with nonorganic hearing loss. Even though it is important for the student in practicum to understand the terms malingering and psychogenic, these terms should not be used in reporting results. It is the audiologist's responsibility to differentiate between organic and nonorganic hearing loss. It is the responsibility of the legal system to determine whether nonorganic hearing loss is malingering. It is the responsibility of psychologists or psychiatrists to diagnose psychogenic origin for nonorganic hearing loss. As the examples presented show, problems often are rooted in the personal and family dynamics.

Central Auditory Processing Problems

Central hearing loss may be divided into two general categories: those with obvious organic causes and those for which an organic cause is not readily identifiable. Regardless of whether an organic cause of central auditory disorder is apparent, all central auditory disorders are manifested in reduced function. What are the primary functions of the central auditory system? The normally functioning central auditory system is capable of:

- **Discriminating** among patterned stimuli. Typically, discrimination is tested by having an individual repeat monosyllabic words.
- **Equal monaural processing.** Equal monaural processing means that messages received at one ear can be understood as well as messages received at the other ear.
- **Binaural processing.** Binaural processing means that messages received in both ears can be understood as well as messages received at either ear.
- **Binaural separation.** When different messages are presented to each of the ears, an individual should be able to attend to one or the other.
- **Binaural summation** and **integration.** When parts of a single message are presented to the two ears, an individual should be able to derive the complete message from the partial information presented to the two ears.
- **Establishing a figure and a ground** from a complex signal. When two or more signals overlap in time and space, an individual should be able to attend to one and to suppress the others.
- **Ordering** sequences of events. An individual should be able to repeat 5 to 9 items in the order in which they were presented.

General Diagnostic Procedures

Evaluation of the central auditory nervous system (CANS) requires a test battery that examines the functions of the auditory system. Many individuals with pure central auditory processing disorders (CAPD) are able to complete most of the tasks required in the peripheral auditory evaluation. However, CAPD reduces the redundancy of central processing for auditory stimuli. When redundancy in the signal (external redundancy) is reduced and presented to a system with reduced internal redundancy, problems arise. Therefore, on such tasks, the individual with CAPD scores much lower than the individual with normal central auditory processing.

Individuals who have CAPD may have more difficulty processing signals at one ear than they do at the other. They may be unable to attend to signals in one or the other ear when competing signals or degraded speech are delivered to the same ear. **Degraded speech** is speech that has been altered to reduce its acoustic redundancy. Speech may be degraded by filtering or by the addition of noise. Individuals with monaural processing problems also may be unable to integrate separate information presented to both ears as well as they can information presented to their better ear alone.

To evaluate binaural processing in an individual with suspected CAPD, tests incorporating dichotic listening tasks are useful. **Dichotic listening tasks** present different but simultaneous signals to each ear. The individual is asked to attend to and report the signal first in one ear and then the other. Dichotic listening tasks will indicate whether the individual being tested has greater difficulty processing auditory signals in one ear as opposed to the other when a competing message is presented to the opposite ear.

The greater difficulty with processing in one ear as opposed to the other ear may be the result of poor processing ability in the poorer ear, or it may be the result of an inability to suppress competing messages in the opposite ear. To find out, compare the results of monaurally presented degraded speech tests to the dichotic task results. By comparing the results of the dichotic tasks with the monaural tasks, it can be determined whether dichotic results were from CAPD in the ear attending to the message or from a lack of suppression in the ear with the competing signal.

When binaural listening tasks provide different signals sequentially at the two ears, and the information from both is required for the individual to perform a task or to identify a message, binaural summation and the integration of the signal from the two ears is needed. It may be useful to compare monaurally presented degraded speech tests to binaurally presented degraded speech tests. If processing of the signal binaurally is worse than would be expected from the monaural scores, difficulty with binaural summation and integration may be suspected.

Speech presented binaurally in a background of noise can be used to evaluate an individual's ability to process information using both ears. If the individual has greater difficulty processing speech in noise received binaurally than he does when speech in noise is received monaurally, it may result from interference of one ear with the other in the binaural listening situation. If monaural performance in noise is better for each ear than the binaural performance, then interference of one ear with the other should be suspected.

Another possible cause of difficulty in processing speech presented binaurally in noise may be an inability of the individual to separate auditory figure from ground. Separating auditory figure from auditory background requires **selective listening.** Selective listening is accomplished by attending to the primary message in one ear while relegating the background noise to the opposite ear and suppressing it. The speech may be filtered, time compressed, or distorted in some other way. Degraded speech presented binaurally does not require selective listening. If binaural scores for speech in noise are worse than scores for spectrally degraded speech material presented binaurally, then binaural separation of signal from background noise should be suspected. It would not be surprising to find that an individual who experiences problems separating auditory figure from auditory ground also has difficulty suppressing a competing message in either or both ears during a dichotic listening task.

An individual may have difficulty recalling a sequence of events, such as digits, when presented auditorily. It is important to make sure that the problem is auditory alone and does not cross modalities. If an individual can visually scan digits and recall them in order, but cannot listen to and repeat back digits, the problem would appear to be specific to the auditory system. If the task cannot be performed either visually or auditorily, the problem would appear to be in short-term memory.

With patterned material, particularly speech, cortical auditory function is assessed. Without intact cortical auditory function, normal auditory processing of speech signals will be impaired. Pattern discrimination requires intact cortical function.

The diagnosis of CAPD is considered advanced diagnosis. Therefore, it is usually covered thoroughly in more advanced graduate courses. The beginning student in audiology practicum is not expected to complete and interpret the results of a CAPD test battery. However, more advanced practicum experiences will include diagnosis of CAPD. Successful management of auditory problems depends on identifying and considering the impact of CAPD. Katz, Stecker, and Henderson (1992); Katz and Wilde (1985); Keith (1981); and Lynn and Gilroy (1984) have presented testing protocols for central auditory processing difficulties.

Causes of Central Auditory Processing Disorders

As stated earlier, CAPD may be found in conjunction with documented organic conditions or exist without documented organic conditions. It is important to recognize organic conditions that may result in CAPD. After consideration of these conditions, CAPD without identifiable organic basis will be discussed.

Organic Disorders Resulting in CAPD

Any number of organic congenital, genetic, and perinatal, postnatal, or later acquired disorders may cause CAPD. The presence of one or more of these factors suggests a need for central auditory processing evaluation. Often, these factors are documented and obviously related to CAPD that result in communicative difficulties. Some of the more common organic causes for CAPD include:

- neoplasams and tumors
- demyelinating diseases, including multiple sclerosis (MS)
- cerebrovascular diseases, including stroke
- degenerative diseases, including Alzheimer's disease
- perinatal and pediatric neuropathology, including various genetic disorders and asphyxia at birth
- infectious and inflammatory diseases, including human immunodeficiency virus (HIV)
- miscellaneous neuropathology
- traumatic head injury

The background and processes of specific diseases under each category and expected effects on auditory responses are readily available in Hall (1992).

CAPD Without Identifiable Organic Cause

There are individuals whose medical and birth histories are unremakable. They have no familial history of nervous system disorders or hereditary conditions that would result in CAPD. They have no history of birth trauma; no history of illness or accident that would account for CAPD. They are of normal or higher intelligence. Yet, these individuals perform poorly on behavioral measures of CAPD. They comprise a unique class of individuals who experience difficulty achieving their potentials. When their communicative environments are appropriately altered, often they are able to function adequately. In schools, these individuals often are labeled as learning disabled and placed in special education classes. As adults, they often are unemployed or work in low paying and unrewarding jobs. Diagnosis can lead to treatment and management resulting in dramatic improvement in their lives and income potential. These individuals often have low motivation and poor self-concepts, but respond to counseling under appropriate circumstances.

We have considered hearing loss by type and discovered that it can be peripheral or central and that peripheral hearing loss is further subdivided into organic and nonorganic types of hearing loss. Organic hearing losses are further subdivided into conductive, sensory, and neural hearing losses. Nonorganic hearing losses may result from malingering behavior or psychogenic causes. Central hearing losses may exist with or without associated, identifiable organic conditions. In addition to type of hearing loss, the amount of the hearing loss affects management strategies. In the next section, diagnosis and quantification of hearing loss will be discussed.

Quantification of Hearing Loss

In audiologic reports summarizing hearing test results, hearing loss is identified by type and amount. Some types of hearing loss indicate certain management strategies and other types, other strategies. Likewise, the amount or quantity of the hearing loss affects the communication difficulty the individual has and, hence, the management strategy to be implemented.

The amount of hearing loss is seldom equal across the frequency spectrum. By far the most common configuration involves greater loss in the high frequencies. Therefore, the terms "high-frequency hearing loss" and "sloping high-frequency hearing loss" are commonly seen in diagnostic reports.

The terms "mild," "moderate," "severe," and "profound" are used to describe organic peripheral hearing loss. These terms are inappropriate for nonorganic hearing loss. With CAPD, the terms "mild, "moderate," and "severe" may be employed. For organic peripheral hearing losses, these terms have very specific definitions. For CAPD, the terms are not specifically defined and represent a judgment of the audiologist. In the following sections, each classification will be defined and discussed.

The effects of hearing loss on speech discrimination are graphically demonstrated with an articulation index (AI). Figure 10-1 is an AI adapted from Mueller and Killion (1990) which presents the distribution of speech energy for normal conversation superimposed on an audiogram. The ordinate is intensity in dB HL and the abcissa is frequency in Hertz. To adapt this chart to quiet conversation, change 0 dB HL on the ordinate to −20 dB HL and so on, resulting in 50 dB HL on the normal conversational level graph becoming the 20 dB HL of quiet conversational level. To adapt the graph of normal conversational levels to loud conversational levels, 0 dB HL becomes 30 dB HL and so on, with 50 dB HL on the normal conversational level graph becoming 70 dB HL on the loud conversational level graph.

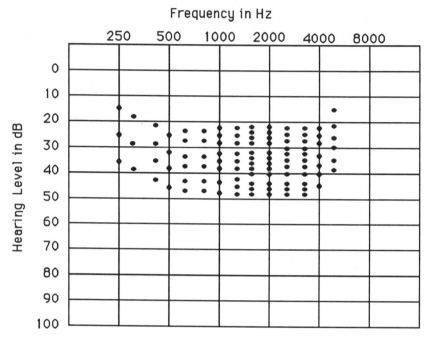

Figure 10-1. An Articulation Index (Speech Inteligibility Index). The distribution of speech energy at normal conversational levels superimposed on the audiogram. From An easy method for calculating the articulation index by H.G. Mueller and M. Killion, 1990, *Hearing Journal, 43*(9), p. 15, adapted by permission.

An individual audiogram may be superimposed and an AI calculated at an appropriate intensity level simply by counting the dots above the individual's threshold curve. There are 100 dots arranged so that the relative weight of each frequency region to intelligibility is accounted for. This representation allows the audiologist to graph the effect of the hearing loss and the effectiveness of the treatment in restoring hearing for speech. In a draft proposal from the ANSI Working Group (1992) standardizing the calculation of the values for the AI, the index has been renamed the Speech Intelligibility Index (SII). Within the next several years, it is expected that the two terms will coexist in practice. At some point in the future, the use of the term SII will replace the term AI. For this discussion the term SII will be used.

To better understand the effects that different amounts of hearing loss have on communication, envision SIIs for quiet, normal, and loud conversation. Normal conversational levels average 50 dB HL. Quiet conversational levels are 20 dB below that level and average 30 dB HL, whereas loud conversational levels are 20 dB above normal conversational levels and average 70 dB HL.

These values represent speech at a distance of 3 feet with the speaker facing the listener. When the speaker is facing away from the listener or is at a distance greater than 3 feet, significant reductions in sound levels occur.

Notice that, under ideal conditions, at quiet conversational levels, the higher frequency consonant sounds are less than 20 dB HL. At normal conversational levels, they are 30 to 40 dB HL, and at loud conversational levels they are 50 to 60 dB HL. Now, imagine that the speaker is a teacher who talks in normal conversational tones but has turned his or her back to the class to write on the chalk board. Also, picture a student sitting in the back row of the class, some 30 feet away from the teacher. At that student's ear, the teacher's voice may be closer to a quiet conversational level.

Mild Hearing Loss

Mild peripheral hearing loss does not exceed 40 dB HL. The level at which mild hearing loss begins may be 15 dB HL for the elementary student, or 25 dB HL for the adult employed in industry. Under commonly accepted medico-legal definitions, hearing loss does not begin until hearing levels exceed 25 dB HL. For medico-legal purposes, the term "mild hearing loss" should not be used for hearing levels better than 25 dB HL.

Medico-legal definitions of normal hearing specify levels between −10 dB and 25 dB HL. However, research has shown that children with hearing levels between 15 and 25 dB HL perform less well than children with hearing between 0 and 15 dB HL (Davis et al., 1986; Quigley, 1968; Ross & Giolas, 1978).

If we return to the example of our student and impose 25 dB HL hearing level over an SII graph adapted to quiet conversation, we can see that the student misses significant numbers of speech sounds. See Figure 10-2 for this configuration of hearing loss imposed on an SII for quiet conversational speech. For the audiologist treating a specific individual, it is important to determine how sensitive the individual's hearing must be to communicate effectively in each situation in which the individual operates. For treatment purposes, the term "mild hearing loss" may be used for hearing levels below 25 dB HL when the individual experiences difficulty hearing.

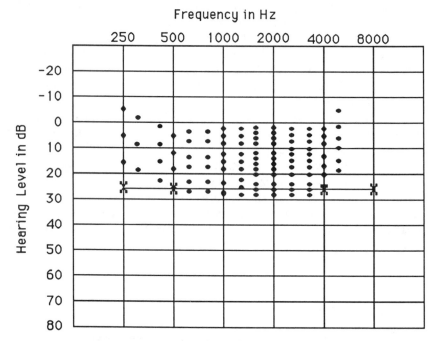

Figure 10-2. The effect, as measured by the SII of a mild hearing loss on the reception of quiet conversational speech. The bilateral hearing loss is symbolized with an X at 25 dB HL. From An easy method for calculating the articulation index by H.G. Mueller and M. Killion, 1990, *Hearing Journal, 43*(9), p. 15, adapted by permission.

For most people, hearing sensitivity worse than 25 dB results in significant hearing problems that interfere with the communication required for daily living. Observe in Figure 10-2 that a hearing level of 25 dB superimposed on quiet conversational speech levels results in a significant number of speech sounds falling below the individual's hearing level. For some elderly individuals who have limited communicative needs, a mild hearing loss of 35 dB HL may cause few communicative or social problems. However, once hearing levels exceed 35 dB HL (mild hearing loss), significant hearing problems exist that affect communicative effectiveness in a great many listening situations.

When the term "mild" is used with CAPD, it indicates that in the audiologist's judgment the CAPD is having significant effects on the communication of the individual. The significant effects, however, do not require the individual to alter his or her lifestyle or change life plans. For example, the individual may not have to quit his or her job or forego favorite activities.

Moderate Hearing Loss

Moderate peripheral hearing loss includes the range of hearing loss between 41 and 70 dB HL. Moderate hearing loss results in significant hearing difficulty and obvious communication problems. If the hearing loss is not treated, the individual may be forced to change his or her lifestyle and alter life plans. An example is a minister with a hearing loss sloping from moderate to severe, acquired after he began his career. He was an excellent communicator and functioned adequately for several years. His lifelong goal was to serve in the mission field, which required that he learn another language. To learn another language he had to be able to hear the sounds basic to that language. Without appropriate amplification to correct for his hearing loss, he would not have been able to hear and acquire the sounds of the language he needed to learn to realize his goal of work in the mission fields.

If we return to the example used before of the student in the classroom and impose 60 dB HL hearing on the SII for normal conversational levels, we can see that the student misses all speech sounds. See Figure 10-3 for this configuration of hearing imposed on the SII for normal conversational speech. When hearing levels exceed 40 dB HL, significant hearing problems exist that affect communication and often the health and welfare of the person.

When the term "moderate" is used with CAPD, it indicates that in the audiologist's judgment the CAPD is having significant effects on the communication of the individual that, unless treated, will require the individual to alter his or her lifestyle or change life plans.

Severe Hearing Loss

Severe peripheral hearing loss includes the range of hearing loss between 71 and 90 dB HL. Severe hearing loss results in significant hearing difficulty and regular and frustrating communication problems. If children with severe hearing loss are not identified early and treated appropriately, development of normal speech and language will be delayed. If acquired severe hearing loss is not treated, individuals will be forced to change their lifestyles and alter their life goals and plans.

If we impose the audiogram of an individual with a severe hearing loss of 80 dB HL on the SII adapted to loud conversation speech, we can see that the individual misses all speech sounds. The individual cannot understand speech shouted from a distance of 3 feet by a speaker facing him or her.

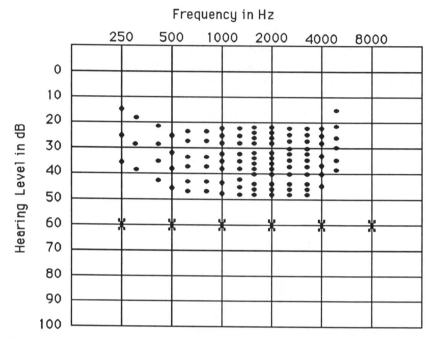

Figure 10-3. The effect, as measured by the SII, of a moderate hearing loss on the reception of normal conversation speech. The bilateral hearing loss is symbolized with an X at 60 dB HL. From An easy method for calculating the articulation index by H.G. Mueller and M. Killion, 1990, *Hearing Journal, 43*(9), p. 15, adapted by permission.

When the term "severe" is used with CAPD, it indicates that in the audiologist's judgment, the CAPD is having significant effects on the communication of the individual that may require the person to alter his or her life plan, even with effective management.

Profound Hearing Loss

Profound peripheral hearing loss includes the range of hearing loss above 90 dB HL. Profound hearing loss results in inability to communicate without appropriate treatment. It is at this level that the term "hearing-impaired" adds the category "deaf." The term "hearing-impaired" refers to anyone with a hearing loss. The term "deaf" refers to a person whose hearing loss is so profound that acquisition of oral language is not possible without intense special educational methods.

Not all individuals with profound hearing losses are classified as deaf. Some can benefit significantly from hearing aids and are capable of effective oral-aural communication. Many are able to achieve effective oral-aural communication with cochlear implants. The term "profound" is not used with CAPD.

In this chapter, diagnosis of auditory disorders of the peripheral and central hearing systems have been discussed. In Chapter 11, a strategy for communicative needs assessment will be examined.

11

Communicative Needs Assessment

Communication problems resulting from hearing loss often are not due to the hearing loss alone. Other factors contribute to those problems. Some of these other factors include the following:

- The client's perceived communication difficulty
- The client's acceptance of communication difficulty
- Listening environments in which the client experiences difficulty
- The client's attitudes and communicative strategy.

The client's **communicative needs assessment** must include evaluation of these factors. Communicative needs assessment develops a profile of how an individual functions. To base management strategies on the results of hearing tests alone increases the risk of mismanagement. Therefore, audiologic evaluation becomes only a part of an overall communicative needs assessment. Under this approach, hearing loss is evaluated for the purpose of defining its effect on the individual's communicative effectiveness, lifestyle, and personal goals.

Preparing to deliver services is as important a process as the actual delivery of services to the client. The following sections will discuss data neededto service the client effectively and methods of obtaining, interpreting, and using the data. Clients often are unable to describe their communicative needs and how their hearing loss affects those needs. Therefore, input from significant others is needed for a more meaningful communicative needs assessment.

It is important that significant others accompany clients to the initial diagnostic session. Adult clients should invite spouses and, in some cases, children. Children should be accompanied by both parents when possible.

Clients are referred or present themselves for services because of perceived difficulty with communication. They may acknowledge having a hearing loss. They may even acknowledge that it causes problems in communication. Clients may focus on hearing loss as the major or even the sole cause of any difficulty that they acknowledge. Many clients, however, do not acknowledge that they have a significant hearing loss. These persons, who believe that they do not have a hearing problem, often give credit to their spouses' insistence for their visit to the audiologist. Frequently, they comment that people mumble and that they can hear well when others speak up. Many times, clients acknowledge hearing loss but deny that it has any effect on their communication or lifestyle. Few people with mild hearing losses are aware of its effect on their ability to communicate. As hearing loss increases, their communicative needs become more obvious.

In environments that are not very demanding on hearing, the client with mild hearing loss may function without perceived difficulty. In other listening environments, great demands are placed on hearing and the client with mild hearing loss perceives difficulty. It is important to determine areas or situations in which difficulty is perceived and whether the client's perceived difficulty matches the actual difficulty. The audiologist's goal is not only to quantify and qualify hearing loss, but to help clients overcome some of their communicative difficulties and to adapt to others.

A communicative needs assessment may be conducted before the audiometric testing commences, or immediately after. Because the client counseling should be based on needs assessment as well as the audiometric results, needs assessment must precede in-depth counseling regarding management strategies.

For many experienced audiologists, the only formal assessment of communicative needs other than the audiometric evaluation is the general case history form. These case histories often are filled out prior to scheduling clients and contain information important to clinical administrative needs. They often reveal only very general information about the client's communicative difficulties.

Many experienced audiologists assess clients' communicative needs in greater detail through informal questioning and incorporate the information gained into their recommendations. In practicum settings where observations of communicative needs are informal, the student should take careful notes on those observations.

The student in practicum and the new clinician in his or her Clinical Fellowship Year are often required to assimilate procedures that may later become an informal part of the evaluation process. New procedures are best learned through formal evaluation, however.

Formal evaluation of a client's communicative needs is required when: (1) the clinic procedures are complex and the new student is overwhelmed by them and (2) the diagnostic situation is complex and requires assimilating and interpreting subtle information. Under these circumstances, it is best for the practicum student to formalize the evaluation of the client's communication needs. A **performance profile** is a graphic presentation of the results of a client's needs assessment and can provide the clinician with an overview of the client's communicative needs.

Determining a Performance Profile

Many tools are available for formal assessment of clients' communication difficulty. The tools used should answer the following questions:

- Does the person perceive difficulty hearing?
- Does the person accept his or her hearing loss as the cause of hearing problems?
- How does a significant other person assess the client's communication difficulty?
- In what situations does the client have difficulty?
  Personal
  Family
  Social
  Work or School
- How does the client feel about and react to perceived communicative difficulty?

- In the environments where hearing difficulty is experienced, what specific listening situations present problems?
- How much time does the client spend in those situations?

The clinician does not need to be with the client when formal inventories are employed. Inventories can be mailed to the clients to be filled out prior to appointments. Experience reveals that few clients complete inventories prior to their appointments. It also is possible to schedule a client and his or her significant other to report 30 minutes before the scheduled testing time to fill out the inventories. The clinician should greet the client and the accompanying person, present them with the inventories, and make sure the instructions are understood before leaving them to complete the inventories. Inventories will identify environments in which clients and their significant others perceive communication difficulty and give their estimate of the client's reaction to auditory failure.

Inventories may be scored before testing clients. Scoring of inventories can be expedited with overlays or computer scoring programs. Scoring and interpretation of the results of the inventories may be helpful in forming an expectation regarding the audiometric results. If the audiometric results differ significantly from the client's perceived level of difficulty, the reasons should be identified. Reasons for differences between the client's and the significant other person's perceptions of their communicative needs affect management strategies and their timing. How the client accepts hearing loss is basic to acceptance of management. Unidentified situational demands on hearing may influence the level of reported communicative difficulty. Unless identified, client expectations for management may be unmet.

Communicative needs assessment varies depending on the age of the client. Therefore, this assessment needs to be considered separately for adults and children.

Adults

Adults may be able to articulate clearly their perceptions of their communication difficulties. Because their hearing losses often are acquired and may be of recent onset, adults have a baseline of more normal hearing with which to compare their current level of hearing. Often, they are motivated to seek help to avoid giving up jobs and allowing personal relationships to deteriorate. On the other hand, adults can be unaware of the effects of hearing loss on their communication. They can deny hearing loss and project the cause of their communication difficulties on speakers "who mumble." The more mature person is open to working through denial and cooperating with the treatment process.

Evaluation of the perceived hearing difficulty of an adult can reveal much about the demands the environment places on that person's hearing and the difficulties he or she experiences. The amount of time individuals spend in difficult listening situations reflects the relative importance of these situations to their lifestyles and the overall difficulty their hearing loss causes them.

The *Revised Hearing Performance Inventory* (RHPI) (Lamb, Owens, & Schubert, 1983) samples the conditions under which the client perceives difficulty. This 90-question inventory is thorough. The method of response is a semantic differential. Possible responses on the semantic differential are "practically always," "frequently," "about half the time," "occasionally," "almost never," or "does not apply." If your practicum facility does not use a hearing performance inventory, you will find the RHPI reproduced in Appendix D. Other inventories are available and are in many aural rehabilitation textbooks (e.g., Alpiner & McCarthy, 1993; Hull, 1991; Sanders, 1993; and Schow & Nerbonne, 1989). From these inventories, clients' perceptions of how much difficulty they have and how often the difficulties are encountered can be assessed.

Schow and Nerbonne (1982) developed the Self-Assessment of Communication (SAC) and the Significant Other Assessment of Communication (SOAC) (Schow & Nerbonne, 1989). Like the RHPI, these inventories provide an estimate of the frequency with which a particular communication difficulty is experienced. Unlike the 90-question RHPI, the SAC and SOAC are short—10 questions long. If you prefer to administer a screening inventory rather than the more comprehensive instrument, the SAC and SOAC may be found in Appendix E.

Children

Children seldom are able to articulate their perceptions of their communication difficulties clearly. Many have no normal baseline with which to compare their current level of hearing. Often, they do not feel good about themselves because they have experienced repeated failure. Fortunately, their communication difficulties may be inferred from their performance. A variety of tools is available for formal assessment of performance. An **educational performance profile** is an appropriate method of organizing the assessment of the communicative needs of children. Examples of educational profiles are available in many introductory special education textbooks. Regardless of the assessment tools used, the following information should be obtained:

- *Physical development.* Is the child within normal height and weight ranges for his or her age group?
- *Social maturity.* Does the child interact with age-group peers and others in an appropriate manner?
- *Speech and language development.* Is speech and language normal for the child's age group?
- *School performance.* Is the child at grade level on standardized tests?
- *Emotional adjustment.* Is the child capable of positive problem solving at a level appropriate to his or her age group? How does the child relate to peers, to adults, and to others? How does the child handle failure?

A performance profile should be obtained before the initial audiometric testing. The audiologist does not need to administer a test battery, but may obtain results from the child's school or an independent educational evaluation agency. Review of the child's profile and audiometric results may reveal a possible relationship between the child's difficulties and the hearing loss. For example, a child may be performing below grade level. The child may have difficulty attending to the teacher when the teacher is addressing the class, but have little difficulty attending to the teacher in one-on-one instruction. A mild bilateral high-frequency hearing loss or a unilateral hearing loss may cause auditory figure-ground problems in a group situation but not when instruction is given individually. If the audiometric results differ significantly from the client's expected profile, other factors influencing the level of communicative difficulty need to be identified. For example, a child performing below grade level may have hearing within normal limits but be seated by an air conditioner that masks out the teacher's voice.

Evaluating the Client's Acceptance of Communication Difficulty

Persons with hearing impairment experience loss just as surely as persons who lose other physical or sensory functions. They must work through stages of grief, as they would for any other loss. Without help, persons experiencing loss may become stuck in one or another stage while working through the grieving process. Denial is a common stage in which persons with hearing impairment may become stuck. Reasons for denying hearing loss vary with age. For example, children may refuse treatment to avoid appearing different from their classmates; whereas, an adult may refuse treatment in denial of the aging process.

Assessment of an adult client's communication difficulty may have shown that the client does have difficulty communicating effectively. It then becomes important to determine whether the client accepts his or her communication difficulties and is ready to accept treatment.

Inventories such as the SAC and SOAC can be used to assess the degree of clients' acceptance of their hearing losses. This assessment is accomplished by comparing inventories completed by the client with inventories completed about the client by another significant person in the client's life. The RHPI can be filled out on a client by the client's significant other. The same inventories that are administered to the adult client should be administered to the spouse of the client with instructions that the spouse should answer for the client. If the spouse perceives significantly greater or less difficulty resulting from the client's hearing problems than does the client, counseling is indicated. The goals of counseling are to (1) determine how much difficulty truly exists and (2) assist one or both parties to adjust their perceptions to better match reality.

The client may perceive less difficulty than the hearing loss indicates or the spouse perceives. Such a client may not accept his or her communication difficulty. Therefore, the client will have difficulty accepting the full effect of the hearing loss and will not be open to counseling and management.

Assessment of acceptance of the hearing loss and the willingness to accept treatment is important in care of children as well. Children, especially late elementary through high school-age children, are very concerned about not appearing different from their peers. Acceptance of a hearing loss that requires special seating, visible hearing aids, and auditory trainers is often resisted. If asked directly, the child may appear cooperative, only to demonstrate passive resistance to management procedures when they are implemented. Management strategies need to be concentrated in efforts to help the individual accept his or her communication difficulty, recognize its significant effects, and accept management of the hearing loss.

Evaluating Listening Environments

Assessment of situational demands specific to the individuals with hearing impairments and their listening situations requires in-depth probing for details by the audiologist. The demands of clients' specific listening environments must be known before a needs assessment can be completed. The hearing performance inventories give only general information about the clients' listening environments. They were designed to ascertain generally under what conditions the clients perceive difficulty listening. The hearing performance inventories measure subjective impressions of the client. Additional sources may provide information that allows the clinician to rate the difficulty of the client's specific listening environments more objectively. These additional sources may vary by the age of the person with hearing impairment.

Listening is affected by the environment in which the signal is transmitted. It is important to understand the acoustic environment of the adult client. What types and levels of noise occur and how often? How often is the client confronted with multiple speakers? How often does the client experience highly reverberant fields? Is ambient noise constant, or does it vary widely in level? Often these questions can be answered by asking clients to describe their daily activities for a week and asking them to describe those in which they have difficulty in more detail. By asking the clients to describe their activities, a knowledge of the amount of precision listening required of them can be determined.

Listening is affected by the content of the message. Military communications research has shown that certain sound combinations are easier to hear than others. Everyday experience tells us that receiving new and highly technical information in a lecture format is more demanding than receiving a greeting from a spouse of 50 years. The retired senior citizen who has returned to college to complete a degree needs greater sensitivity in hearing than the senior who lives alone, reads, gardens, and rarely leaves home. By questioning clients about their daily activities and how well they perform them, audiologists can estimate the situational demands made on their hearing.

Comparing children's performance profiles and their audiometric results may indicate a relationship between hearing loss and the performance profile. However, in some cases, performance profiles may indicate performance much worse than can be accounted for on the basis of hearing loss alone.

Classroom environments are often noisy and highly reverberant. Children with hearing loss may be located far from the teacher. Obtaining answers to several questions will help evaluate the classroom as a listening environment. Where is the child located relative to the teacher? What are the room's reverberant characteristics? What is the ambient noise level in the room? What is the frequency spectrum of the ambient noise? Answers to these questions suggest classroom management strategies.

Sometimes, children's performance profiles are much better than would be expected on the basis of their hearing. Many children who are hearing impaired learn to give socially acceptable responses that teachers misinterpret as correct answers. Sometimes, teachers recognize a child's hearing loss and reduce requirements or issue grades on the basis of effort rather than mastery of skills or subject matters.

Some very bright and highly adaptable children will have such a large reserve of ability so that they are able to complete work to grade level with little effort. Such children are not as adversely affected by hearing loss as are less talented children.

Even though the classroom often presents the most demanding listening environment by presenting new and perhaps technical information, listening demands can be reduced by student preparation and altering teachers' presentation styles. A review of the child's study habits and the teacher's method of presenting information may provide clues to effective methods for preparation by the child and presentation by the teacher. Also, as with adults, interviewing children, parents, and teachers about daily activities and the amount of difficulty the child has performing them can provide a good estimate of the situational demands on the child's hearing.

Evaluating the Client's Attitudes and Communicative Strategy

Once the client's perceived difficulty, acceptance of his or her hearing loss, and the situational demands on his or her hearing have been evaluated, the appropriateness of the client's attitudes and communication strategy should be assessed. Three areas should be examined more closely.

- Client expectations
- Attitudes of significant others
- Appropriate client response criteria

Client's Expectations

Even if a person recognizes communication difficulty and is open to management, inappropriate expectations for treatment outcomes may undermine the management process. For example, the person who obtains a hearing aid and expects to hear better in noise than does a normal-hearing individual has inappropriate expectations. The clinician should question the client about his or her expectations.

Attitudes of Significant Others

The attitudes of others may affect what an individual expects from treatment. Sometimes the individual's family physician has diagnosed a "nerve deafness" and suggested that a hearing aid will not help. At other times, negative experiences by friends or relatives with improper fittings, inappropriate expectations, or both may create negative dispositions toward the use of a hearing aid. Therefore, the client's perceptions of the expectations of significant others regarding treatment outcomes should be carefully assessed.

If expectations are not realistic, management through counseling to encourage the client to adopt realistic expectations for treatment outcomes is indicated. Part IV will present strategies for counseling clients with inappropriate expectations. Treatment options for hearing loss may need to be delayed until the client expectations are modified.

Appropriate Client Response Criteria

An individual's response to a message detected through the senses is affected by two factors: (1) the sensory ability of the person to analyze and interpret the signal and (2) the criterion the individual chooses for responding. The **criterion for response** depends on knowledge of the context of the message and the payoff matrix for the receiver of the message. The **payoff matrix** weights the costs and gains to the receiver of various response options. For example, a receiver of a message may think, "I am unsure of the signal and, therefore, I may guess the message content wrongly. I cannot be wrong; therefore, I will not respond to the message, but instead will ask the speaker to repeat the message." The appropriateness of the response criterion given in the example depends on whether the actual situation required that the listener be sure of the signal before responding. The speaker may be more irritated by being asked to repeat than by a misunderstood message that the speaker repeats on his or her own initiative. Guessing behaviors reflect response criteria. The appropriateness of response criteria can be plotted as a receiver operating characteristic. Guessing behavior may be quantified to provide a measure of an individual's response criterion in a given situation.

Hearing loss may affect a person's guessing behavior in at least three ways. The person may continue to guess as if he or she heard normally. The person may guess less than he or she did when hearing was normal. The person may begin to guess more than when his or her hearing was normal. Any of these strategies may be appropriate. The measure of their appropriateness is related to how the guessing strategy affects the accuracy of the message perception.

Persons who guess as they did when their hearing was normal may not take the hearing loss into account. Such persons may respond "five o'clock," when asked the question, "Do you have a dime?" They do not recognize the need to ask for clarification when sound confusions are likely. They do not adopt a more conservative criterion for guessing when sound confusions are likely.

Sometimes, people recognize that they have a hearing loss and overreact. Such a person may think, "I cannot hear; therefore, I can only understand the most obviously communicated information. I should not guess, or ask for clarification, but withdraw when communication becomes difficult." A variation on this theme is the person who thinks that, "I cannot hear well enough to understand correctly what the other person is saying; therefore, I will do all the talking." Either way, effective communication is thwarted.

Other persons with hearing impairment increase their guessing behavior beyond available information to the point that their responses are inappropriate to the messages communicated by others. These persons seem to be in a different reality than the one in which everyone else operates. They most often are people to whom it is extremely important to maintain communication and social relationships. They also are the ones most devastated by misunderstanding.

The appropriateness of a client's criterion for responding to a message can be quantified. Using a signal detection paradigm, a measure of the client's sensitivity to signal differences (d') and a measure of the client's criterion for response, Beta (β), can be obtained. These two scores compared to the percent correct score on a speech discrimination task will indicate the appropriateness of the client's response criterion.

Let us say that a particular client scored 60% on the Northwestern University Speech Discrimination Test (NU-6). However, on a paired nonsense syllable, same-different test, the same client scored a high d' and a β score greatly in excess of the ideal. The speech discrimination is poor (60% on the NU-6). The client's ability to discriminate sound is good (a high d'). Guessing behavior is inappropriately conservative (a β score greatly in excess of the ideal). The implications are that the client needs to be trained to change his or her criterion for responding. The criterion should be less stringent. The client should be taught to guess appropriately about the messages he or she hears. Appendix F contains a 50-item same-different nonsense syllable test. Appendix G contains information on deriving and interpreting the d' and β scores for a two-interval, forced-choice test like that found in Appendix F. Once the appropriateness of the client's criterion for response is determined, a decision can be made on how to integrate techniques designed to reinforce appropriate response criteria with management of the hearing loss.

Assessing Other Communication Problems

Audiologists cannot be so myopic that they miss all other types of communication disorders except for hearing loss. In addition to assessing auditory problems and the impact they have on a client, audiologists need to screen for speech production and language problems. The first semester practicum student may be tempted to concentrate on hearing and to ignore the assessment of speech and language. Instead, you need to make a concerted effort to screen each client for speech and language problems and to make the appropriate referrals when necessary.

Assessing Speech and Language Problems

Speech and language production may be screened formally or informally. Informal screening of articulation, voice, language, and fluency can be accomplished by having the client read a passage. The *Rainbow Passage* or *Grandfather Passage* are two examples of connected discourse used for informal assessment of articulation, voice, language, and fluency. These passages are readily available in many speech and language pathology textbooks. An even more informal, and yet quite appropriate, method of screening speech and language is to monitor conversation during the case history interview. Formal screening instruments for articulation, voice, and language are available. As in other areas of assessment, the authors suggest that practicum students formalize procedures. Through the use of formal procedures you learn thoroughness. Later, if you elect to conduct certain procedures informally, you will know the content to include.

An Outline for Auditory Diagnostics

The student in practicum might view diagnosis in audiology as a complex process, and rightfully so. The equipment and procedures available for evaluation of the auditory system have expanded exponentially in the last few years. However, students can organize their approaches to diagnostics and avoid being overwhelmed. An outline containing a series of questions allows systematic elimination of possibilities and leaves the student with tenable conclusions. One must remember that the primary purpose of diagnosis is management and that diagnosis of auditory problems depends less on equipment and more on the skill of the professional audiologist. What you do with the results of your testing is more important than what equipment you have available.

The following outline consists of a series of questions that will guide you through the diagnostic process. Answer them in order and draw appropriate conclusions. Report your conclusions with appropriate qualifiers to your supervisor. With the guidance of your supervisor, you will develop the necessary skills to become proficient in diagnosis of auditory system problems.

Questions

- Who is this person?
  Name?
  Address?
  Age?
  Medical history?
  Employment?
- Why is the person here?
- How does the person perceive the effect of any hearing loss?
  Communication
  Social
  Personal
  School or employment

- What are the environmental demands on the person's hearing?
- What are the person's expectations of the outcome of services?
- What is the person's listening strategy?
- Does the person have a hearing loss?
  Is the hearing loss organic or nonorganic?
  Is the hearing loss peripheral or central?
  If peripheral:
    Conductive?
    Sensory?
    Neural?
    Mixed?
  If central:
    Associated with organic conditions?
    Not associated with organic conditions?
- How much hearing loss is there?
    Mild?
    Moderate?
    Severe?
    Profound?
- What management may be appropriate?
- Would referral for other services be appropriate?

Certainly, there are many acceptable approaches to diagnosis. The outline of questions given here is just one. It is hoped that it will serve you well as you approach diagnostics in practicum.

A few comments are required concerning efficiency in diagnostics. You are **efficient** in diagnostics when you complete the necessary tests and client counseling in the period of time allotted by the facility in which you are located. University training programs often require the student to administer more tests than may be considered necessary, or even prudent, by a hospital, medical, or private practice. University clinics often allow 1 to 2 hours per scheduled patient. Many facilities outside the university setting schedule patients for initial diagnostics in 30 minute blocks.

How much time is appropriate for testing air, bone, speech reception, and speech discrimination? In the university training clinic, 30 to 45 minutes may be required when results for these tests are obtained utilizing conservative techniques, and rightfully so. The student is learning standard techniques. In a fast-paced medical setting, the audiologist may be expected to deliver these results in 20 to 30 minutes, depending on whether the audiologist is expected to inform the client about the results.

Time can be saved in several ways when doing air, bone, and speech reception testing. For instance, you may estimate hearing levels and present model tones at 10 dB above the estimated levels, instead of always beginning at 30 dB HL and searching from that level. Instead of rechecking 1000 Hz for reliability for each ear and by air- and bone-conduction, the recheck may be performed once. Also, instead of completing an entire threshold procedure during the recheck, the tone can be presented 10 dB below the previously acquired response and increased in 5 dB steps. If the client responds within 5 dB of the previous response, you have established reliability. When masking, instead of using minimal levels and increasing the noise in 5 dB increments, increase the noise in 10 to 20 dB increments, being cautious not to overmask. When the two ears are equal by air conduction and the first bone-conduction test is not different than the air-conduction thresholds, treat that as a common bone-conduction result and do not test the other ear by bone conduction. As you demonstrate mastery of standard techniques and gain confidence, your supervisors will suggest other time-saving techniques.

One of the most time-consuming problems associated with diagnosis occurs when clients are allowed to interrupt the diagnostic process by visiting. Many older persons, in particular, are lonely and will take advantage of an opportunity to socialize. Sometimes it is difficult to remain on task and to maintain rapport at the same time. This clinical skill comes with practice. If you have difficulty in this area, ask your supervisor for guidance.

Diagnosis of auditory problems is part of the overall assessment of communicative needs which has the purpose of identifying management options and guiding choice among those options. Part IV will examine management options and develop a strategy for delivering services.

Part IV

Management of Problems Related to Hearing Loss

The previous section outlined a diagnostic strategy to identify clients' communicative needs associated with hearing loss. Communicative needs assessment provides the basis for management of communicative problems related to hearing loss. Several excellent texts deal with the management of persons with hearing-related problems (Alpiner & McCarthy 1993; Hull, 1992; Sanders, 1993; Sandlin, 1990; Schow & Nerbonne, 1989.) It is not the purpose of Part IV to duplicate the information found in other sources. Rather, its purpose is to introduce students to a problem-solving strategy for approaching management problems that are commonly encountered in practicum, but not well delineated in text books. Effective clinical management results from correctly identifying and solving problems.

Diagnosis of hearing loss and related communication problems has two purposes: to reduce the **health risk** of active medical pathology associated with hearing loss and to reduce **communication problems** of persons with hearing losses. Sometimes, solving the problems related to hearing loss is straightforward; at other times, solving them is complicated by other factors. Problems will be addressed in the order in which they are likely to be encountered in the management process. Before presenting specific problems, an outline of general options available for management of hearing problems will be presented. **Audiologic management** refers to the specific services provided by an audiologist within the general options for management of problems related to hearing loss. Some audiologic management procedures reduce health risks; most reduce communication problems.

General Options for Management of Hearing Problems

The following four areas should be considered in managing a person with a hearing loss:

- Medical/surgical treatment
- Hearing aids
- Techniques to modify communicative behavior
- Techniques to modify social, psychological, vocational, or educational aspects of the client's existence.

Provision of these services may take place independently, but they often overlap in most management plans. As a student in practicum, you may expect to be involved in audiologic management in all these areas.

Part IV is organized into four chapters, one for each of the major management categories. Problems to be solved are stated, followed by solutions, and specific step-by-step problem-solving procedures when thought to be helpful. Complicating factors are listed and, if applicable, briefly discussed.

12

Audiologic Management Related to Medical or Surgical Treatment

Audiologic management may include cerumen removal, referral for medical or surgical evaluation and treatment, and pre- and post-medical or surgical management. The diagnostic process may reveal problems to be solved before diagnostics can be completed and other management options considered.

In otoscopic examination of an ear canal, an accumulation of cerumen can obscure your view of the tympanic membrane. In addition, an excessive accumulation of cerumen can preclude obtaining an adequate earmold impression. Further, impacted cerumen can cause significant conductive hearing loss.

Problem 12-1. The client presents with an excessive accumulation of cerumen.
Solution 12-1. Remove the cerumen.

Procedure for Cerumen Removal

Step 1. Examine the ear canal with an otoscope.
- Determine that the obstructing material is cerumen.
- Since the tympanic membrane cannot be viewed because of cerumen, review the audiogram and immittance test results to determine whether either of the following exists:
  1. Inability to maintain a seal during immittance testing.
  2. A flat pressure-compliance function and high physical volume.

  These conditions indicate that the middle ear may be accessible through the ear canal and require medical referral. If there is no indication of a hole in the tympanic membrane, proceed to step 3.

Step 2. Ask the client the following questions:
- Do you have P.E. tubes in your ear?
- Have you had an earache recently?
- Have you had ear surgery?
- Does this ear drain?
- Have you experienced dizziness recently?
- Are you diabetic?
- Do you have AIDS?
- Do you have any other possible condition that may put you at risk with this procedure?

  A "yes" answer to any of these questions indicates a need for **medical referral.** "No" answers to these questions enable you to proceed to step 3.

Step 3. Re-examine the ear canal with an otoscope. Note the size, shape, and general direction of the ear canal and estimate the location of the tympanic membrane.

Step 4. Explain the procedure to the client and obtain his or her informed consent by asking permission to proceed.

Step 5. Soften the cerumen.
- Inform the client that the softing process takes a minimum of 30 to 45 minutes and may require repeated applications.
- Have the client lie on his or her side, or sit in a position to tilt the head with the ear containing the cerumen up to contain liquid.
- Place a **cerumenolytic,** carbamide peroxide (6.5%) and glycerin, in the ear canal. Wait 30 to 45 minutes.

Step 6. Irrigate the ear canal.
* Seat the client in an upright position.
* Place a plastic sheet or a towel on the client's upper body to protect his or her clothing.
* Have the client hold an **emesis basin,** a kidney-shaped bowl, against the side of the neck just below the ear to catch water as it runs out of the ear. The client's head should be tilted slightly downward toward the basin. Additional towels should be available to dry the side of the client's face and neck, if necessary.
* Fill the irrigator basin with tap water at body temperature, 37° centigrade.
* Set the irrigator at a low setting. The stream of water should appear steady rather than obviously pulsating. Higher pressures are not necessary to dislodge cerumen and can be uncomfortable and cause damage to the ear. Purge the water from the tip and hose before irrigating the ear to avoid flushing the ear with cool water which may cause dizziness.
* Straighten the client's ear canal by pulling upward and back on the superior portion of the pinna.
* Place the tip of the irrigator into the ear canal so that the stream of water will be directed superiorly. Do not block the ear canal with the irrigator tip, because the stream will build up a slight pressure behind the impacted cerumen, break it up, and then drain out the inferior portion of the canal along with fragments of the ear wax.
* Place your hand or forearm against the side of the client's head to prevent damage to the ear by movement of the client's head.
* Allow the client to push the button controlling the pump. The client should feel free to push the button off at anytime during the process.
* Irrigate the ear for approximately 30 seconds.

Step 7. Re-examine the ear canal with an otoscope. If the ear canal is clear and the tympanic membrane visible, you are finished irrigating the canal. Go to step 10. If there is loose debris in the ear canal, go to step 8. If large amounts of cerumen are still present, repeat steps 5, 6, and 7. If cerumen is present after repeating the procedure, go to step 8.

Step 8. Remove the debris. A **cerumen spoon,** a blunt ear curette or wire curette, may be used to remove chunks of cerumen dislodged but not washed out during irrigation. Use good light, do not penetrate deeply, and do not scrape the ear canal surface. The ear canal surface is very delicate and may lacerate and bleed, causing the client discomfort. If the ear canal is now clear of cerumen and the tympanic membrane visible, go to step 9. Removal of the cerumen often results in a reddening of the ear canal and tympanic membrane. You should not be alarmed. If cerumen is still visible in the ear canal, complete steps 9, 10, and 11. It should be noted that some practitioners prefer to use curettes as a first step, suction as a second step, and irrigation as a last step. This preference is currently taught in the cerumen management course sponsored by the American Academy of Dispensing Audiologists.

Step 9. If no bleeding is observed, place several drops of 70% alcohol solution into the ear canal with the client's head tilted so that the alcohol remains in the ear for a few seconds.
• Have the client straighten his or her head, allowing any remaining liquid to drain away.
• Re-examine the ear canal with an otoscope to make sure that the ear canal is free of fluid.

Step 10. Document the activity on the client's chart.

Step 11. Reschedule the client.
• Provide the client with a cerumenolytic.
• Instruct the client to apply it to the ear canal twice daily for four days prior to his or her next clinic visit.
• At the next scheduled visit, repeat steps 5 and 6. If cerumen still remains in the ear in amounts sufficient to obscure the tympanic membrane, complete steps 9 and 10 and make a **medical referral.**
    Several commercially available over-the-counter ear wax removal kits include a carbamide peroxide solution and an ear syringe for flushing the ear canal, so that clients may, by periodic application, prevent excessive accumulation and impaction of cerumen.

Complicating Factors
When wax is impacted in the ear canal, it must be removed. The removal of impacted earwax can be easy or complicated.

Factor 1. The difficulty of removal. When wax adheres to the earcanal wall, is extremely dense, or combines with hair to provide a very strong barrier resistant to removal, the process of removal becomes more involved and requires special instrumentation.

Factor 2. Tympanic membrane perforation. When there is a strong possibility that tympanic membrane may be perforated, the chances of exposing the middle ear to fluid and debris from the ear canal are increased.

Factor 3. Special medico-legal prohibitions. Even though ASHA has defined cerumen removal as within the scope of audiologic practice, some states may have legal opinions from attorneys for the Medical Board defining cerumen removal as a medical practice and limiting cerumen removal to physicians or employees directly under their supervision.

Factor 4. Supervisor preference. Even when cerumen removal is legally within the scope of practice of audiologists, some audiologists may not have been trained to remove cerumen or prefer not to remove cerumen.

These factors complicate cerumen removal by introducing an extra step in the procedure: referral' to a physician. Referral for cerumen removal is best made to the specialist who has the appropriate illuminating and magnifying devices, suction devices, and instruments to remove the cerumen with the least trauma to the ear canal. The audiologist or physician without this specialized equipment should avoid probing in the ear. To do so may cause laceration to the canal or the ear drum and a great deal of discomfort for the client.

The audiologist must be aware of conditions that may require medical or surgical treatment. Whenever any of the following conditions are observed, hearing-impaired persons should be advised that it is in their best interest to consult a physician, preferably one who specializes in the diseases of the ear:

- Visible congenital or traumatic deformity of the ear
- Active drainage, or a history of drainage, from the ear within the past 3 months
- A history of sudden or rapidly progressive hearing loss within the past 3 months
- Unilateral hearing loss of sudden or recent onset within the past 3 months
- Acute or chronic dizziness
- A significant air-bone gap.

Problem 12-2. The client presents with a condition that requires medical referral.
Solution 12-2. Refer the client for otologic consultation.

Procedure for Referral to a Physician

Step 1. Inform the client that he or she may have an active medical problem and that it is in his or her best interest to see a physician, preferably one who specializes in diseases of the ear. Inform the client of the reason for the referral. State the observation that you made that resulted in the referral.

Step 2. Encourage the client to ask any questions he or she has and answer them succinctly.

Step 3. Ask the client to request that a report from the physician be sent to the clinic.

Step 4. Encourage the client to return for follow-up testing after medical evaluation and treatment, if indicated. This will help you maintain client contact to assess the client's need for additional services.

Complicating Factors
Any time a client is referred elsewhere for services, there is a possibility that you will lose control of the client's management process. Always refer to physicians who send reports in a timely fashion, appreciate your services, and refer the client back to you.

Factor 1. The physician to whom the client is referred does not report his or her diagnosis and treatment to the clinic. Without this information, you may not be able to follow-up with your client. Telephone your client within 2 to 3 weeks of the referral to determine whether he or she followed up on your referral and, if the client did, whether the physician was asked to send a report to you. If the client saw the physician, requested a report, and it has been 2 weeks or more since the visit, telephone the physician's office and request the report.

Factor 2. After seeing the physician, the client does not return to you for audiologic management. The client may have received misinformation and may not seek further management. Sometimes the physician tells the client that nothing can be done for a "nerve" hearing loss, indicating that there is no effective medical or surgical treatment option. The client may interpret this to mean that options other than medical treatment or surgery will not be effective and, as a result, seeks no further management.

Referral of a client for medical management does not preclude the need for continued audiologic management. Otitis media, otosclerosis, and unaidable profound sensorineural hearing loss are three conditions in which audiologic management, in concert with otologic management, may be beneficial. In addition, intraoperative monitoring is a form of audiologic management that compliments otologic management. Therefore, in the following sections, problems associated with audiologic management of clients with otitis media will be presented first. Next, audiologic management of clients with otosclerosis and unaidable profound sensorineural hearing loss will be discussed. Finally, intraoperative monitoring will be introduced and the practicum student's role clarified.

Otitis media is infection in the middle ear. Its beginning stages often are marked by malfunctioning eustachian tubes. The mucous membrane that lines the middle ear absorbs air. Unless the eustachian tube functions properly, the eardrum becomes severely retracted and the middle ear space fills with fluid. The client initially presents with negative pressure-compliance functions less than -200 decapascal (daPa). In advanced stages, the middle ear fills with fluid, and the pressure-compliance function flattens.

Problem 12-3. The client has significantly negative middle ear pressure. Solution 12-3. Attempt to equalize the middle ear pressure.

Procedure to Equalize Middle Ear Air Pressure

Step 1. The question is whether the eustachian tube functions well enough to equalize the pressure. Inform the client that you will have him or her perform an exercise or two that may equalize the air pressure in the middle ear with the air pressure in the ear canal. The first procedure is the **Toynbee procedure,** which involves having the client pinch the nares closed and holding the mouth closed while swallowing. If that procedure does not open the eustachian tube and allow air pressure to balance between the middle ear and ear canal, a second procedure will be completed. The second procedure is the **Valsalva procedure** which involves having the client pinch the nares closed while closing the mouth and blowing hard. Ask the client if he or she wishes to proceed.

Step 2. Administer the Toynbee procedure.
- Ask the client to close his or her mouth.
- Have the client gently pinch his or her nares closed with the thumb and forefinger.
- Instruct the client to swallow. A sip of water held in the mouth may be used to facilitate swallowing, if necessary.

Step 3. Re-administer immittance and observe changes in the pressure-compliance function. If pressure-compliance has shifted positively, you have determined the eustachian tube for that ear to be functional, and you may terminate the procedure. If negative air pressure in the middle ear is still in excess of −200 daPa, go to step 4.

Step 4. Administer the Valsalva procedure.
- Ask the client to close his or her mouth.
- Have the client gently pinch his or her nares closed with the thumb and forefinger.
- Instruct the patient to blow.
- Repeat step 3. If air pressure is greater than +50 daPa, read-minister step 2. If air pressure does not change, step 4 may be repeated. If after two repetitions of step 4 there remains significantly negative air pressure remains in the middle ear, reschedule the client for repeat eustachian tube evaluation.

Complicating Factors

Negative middle ear pressure may indicate a temporary condition or it represent the beginning of otitis media.

Factor 1. Acute otitis media may develop between appointments. The client should be advised that this is a possiblity and that he or she immediately should seek medical treatment if ear pain or hearing loss occurs.

Factor 2. Excessive positive pressure may result from the Valsalva procedure. In a few instances, the client may experience discomfort that is not relieved by repeated Toynbee procedures. Medical referral to an ear specialist and eustachian tube inflation may be necessary.

When the ear fills with fluid, ear pain and hearing loss may result. The conservative medical treatment for otitis media is an antibiotic for infection and an antihistamine-decongestant to restore eustachian tube function and clear the middle ear of fluid. If conservative medical treatment does not work and chronic otitis media results, surgery may be indicated. **Chronic otitis media** is a condition that does not respond to treatment over an extended period of time. The surgery may consist of adenoidectomy and transtympanic tube implantation, or tube implantation alone.

It is imperative that individuals receiving surgical management for otitis media be monitored audiologically. Implanted tubes must remain in place and patent long enough to allow the eustachian tube to restore normal functioning.

Problem 12-4. The transtympanic tube appears blocked and nonfunctional with a flat pressure-compliance function.
Solution 12-4. Determine whether the tube is patent.

Procedure to Determine Whether Tubes are Patent

Step 1. Inform the client that you are going to place +200 daPa air pressure in his or her ear and observe the client's ability to retain a seal. Obtain the client's permission to proceed.

Step 2. Introduce +200 daPa pressure into the ear canal and observe the air-pressure indicator. A quick return of pressure toward 0 dapa indicates a patent tube. A physical volume measured in excess of 2.5 cc for an adult also indicates a patent tube. If the physical volume of the ear canal measured is below 1.5 cc for the adult or 1.0 cc for the child, or the quick return of air pressure from +200 daPa to 0 daPa does not occur, the client should be referred back to the surgeon with the recommendation that the tube be cleared. After referral to the surgeon, the client should be reevaluated.

Complicating factors
Postsurgical maintenance of transtympanic tube implacement has not been common, except in rare instances of secondary infection. The surgeon may be reluctant to attempt removal of cerumen from a blocked tube.

Factor 1. Anesthesia may be required with its inherent risks. The surgeon may think the risks associated with anesthesia outweigh the benefit of a patent tube.

Factor 2. Without anesthesia, surgical risks are increased. The surgeon may think the risks of suctioning cerumen from an implanted tube without anesthesizing the patient outweigh the benefit of a patent tube.

Problem 12-5. With transtympanic tube implacement, water may enter the middle ear.
Solution 12-5. Provide custom swimmer's ear molds.

Procedure for Providing Custom Swimmer's Ear Molds
Even though the surgeon may have warned them against getting water in their ears, clients with transtympanic tube implantation. bathe, use spas, and swim. Custom-made swimmer's ear plugs will prevent water from accumulating in the ear. Such plugs are a treatment option best supplied by the audiologist. They are ordered from earmold manufacturers. Manuals provided by earmold manufacturers give detailed instructions on obtaining good earmold impressions and ordering swimmer's ear plugs.

Problem 12-6. The client does not know how to use and care for the swim plugs.
Solution 12-6. Provide orientation in the care and use of swim plugs.

Procedure for Orientation in the Care and Use of Swimmer's Ear Plugs

Step 1. Instruct the client when to use the ear plugs.
• Insert the ear plugs prior to entering the swimming pool.
• Insert the ear plugs prior to entering the spa.
• Insert the ear plugs prior bathing.

Step 2. Instruct the client on the insertion and removal of the ear plugs.
• Instruct the patient to straighten the ear canal by reaching behind the head with the opposite hand and gently pulling up and back on the posterior-superior portion of the pinna.
• With the swim plug tab positoned between the client's thumb and index finger of the hand on the side of the head into which the plug is to be inserted, align the canal portion of the ear plug so that it is angled pointing slightly forward.
• Have the client push the ear plug into the ear canal with a slight twisting motion until it is seated properly. Have the client remove his or her hand from the ear and observe the inserted plug. A properly seated swimmer's ear plug will fill the concha, feel comfortable but snug, and attenuate sound slightly.
• Direct the client to grasp the tab of the plug and pull the plug from the ear. A slight twisting motion while pulling may ease removal.

- Complete this procedure with each ear. Repeat this step a minimum of three times per ear or until you are satisfied the client can insert and remove the plugs with ease.

Step 3.   Instruct the client in the care of the ear plugs.
- Swimmer's ear plugs should be rinsed in warm tap water to remove chlorine after use in swimming pools and spas.
- Ear plugs should not be left in the sun or placed near a heater.
- As needed, the ear plugs should be cleaned in warm water containing a small amount of mild liquid dish washing soap. The plugs should be dried thoroughly before replacing them in the ears. Alcohol should not be used to clean the plugs because it will dry and harden them.

Complicating Factor

Swimmer's ear plugs come out while the client is in the water. Ear plugs that become dislodged in swimming pools can be lost and may damage filtering systems. Properly designed swimmer's ear plugs will float to the surface and can be retrieved easily. However, the client may get water in the ear unless the plug is wiped off and reseated before water is introduced into the ear.

The danger of dislodging a swimmer's plug is greater with children at play. Careful instruction to the client to dry the plug and reinsert it is necessary. Children at play in a pool should be carefully supervised. If an accident occurs so that water enters the postsurgical ear, the client should see the surgeon.

As can be seen in the preceding discussion, audiologic management options compliment medical and surgical treatment options for otitis media. Audiologic management options for other conditions also compliment otologic treatment for those conditions.

Otosclerosis is a disease process that may result in the fixation of the ossicular chain. The area of the chain most often affected is where the footplate of the stapes fits into the oval window. Another area affected is the incudostapedial joint. **Ankylosis,** calcium deposits in joints reducing their mobility, results in conductive hearing loss. With the fixation of the ossicular chain, greater hearing loss by bone conduction at 2000 Hz may be observed than at other frequencies. When the fixation is at the incudostapedial joint, a high-frequency air-bone gap is observed. The progress of the disease may be slowed or arrested by medical treatment that centers around regulation of calcium absorption. Hearing can be restored only with surgery. However, hearing aids may compensate for the loss and often are needed even with successful surgery. Hearing aids are an alternative for clients for whom surgery is not an option.

When sensory hearing loss results in unaidable profound hearing loss, a cochlear implant is a management option. Determining candidacy for and successful management of cochlear implants requires a team approach. A surgeon implants the device. The audiologist manages the programming of the implant and training of the client to make maximal use of the resultant sensations. Specialized training for the programming of an implant device is conducted by the manufacturers of the various devices. Students in an advanced off-campus placement that provides cochlear implant services may be instructed in the programming of the device by his or her supervisor. Training in the use of the device is well covered in Mecklenberg (1990). A case study of acquired deafness and cochlear implant management is presented in Nerbonne, Smedley, Tannahill, Schow, and Flevaris-Phillips (1989).

When surgery to remove an VIIIth nerve tumor is a treatment option, intraoperative monitoring by an audiologist may be requested. A licensed and experienced audiologist may seek special training in order to offer this service. It would be unusual for a student in training to participate in intraoperative monitoring.

When medical or surgical management of hearing loss does not restore hearing to normal levels, hearing aids are an appropriate management tool. Chapter 13 follows with a discussion of management strategies involving hearing aids.

13

Audiologic Management with Amplification

Audiologic management includes provision of hearing aids, assistive listening devices, and related services. Clients with conductive, sensory, and neural hearing losses may be candidates for amplification.

As mentioned before, a client with otosclerosis may elect amplification as an alternative to surgery. Some conditions that may influence a client to elect amplification over surgery are advanced age, poor general health, or a specific health condition that increases the risk of surgery. Also, amplification alone may reduce the effects of the hearing loss as effectively as a combination of surgery and amplification.

Amplification may be a temporary remedy for conductive hearing loss resulting from otitis media until surgery becomes an acceptable alternative. For example, a child with a moderate conductive hearing loss, because of poor general physical and emotional health resulting from physical abuse, was required to wait a year for surgery. In the meantime, she had to communicate in her foster home and at school. Amplification provided a temporary remedy for this child's communication problems until her health allowed surgery to restore her hearing.

Sensory hearing loss results from a variety of causes. Noise-induced hearing loss and presbyacusis are the two most common causes of sensory hearing loss. Neither condition is classified as active pathology. Meniere's disease, on the other hand, may signal a medically or surgically treatable condition. Meniere's disease requires thorough medical evaluation and treatment, if indicated. However, sensory hearing loss, including that resulting from Meniere's disease, is most effectively managed through amplification. As discussed in Chapter 11, candidacy for amplification is determined by the client's hearing loss, listening needs, and attitude toward amplification.

Hearing Aids

Procedures for hearing aid evaluation and the selection are discussed in many sources (Katz, 1985; Martin, 1991; Sandlin, 1988, 1990). Selection procedures vary. Students in practicum facing their first hearing aid selection often are overwhelmed by the variety of procedures available and need specific solutions for solving problems encountered.

Problem 13-1. Selecting the appropriate type of hearing aid.

Solution 13-1. Select the full concha in-the-ear (ITE) unless otherwise indicated.

Complicating Factors
Full concha ITE hearing aids provide dispensers with the greatest ability to customize the hearing aid to the user with a full range of optional adjustments available. Severe and greater hearing loss, patient preferences, and limited special features on some hearing aids complicate the choice of hearing aid type.

Factor 1. Power output requirements. Severe-to-profound hearing loss requires more powerful amplification than is available in most ITE instruments. Even ITE instruments considered to be powerful are limited by feedback, because of the close proximity of the microphone and speaker in the ITE instrument. Tight-fitting shells with extended canals and soft tips have extended the range of ITE fittings on some clients to 80 dB HL. A development first introduced in 1993 by one hearing aid manufacturer senses and controls feedback with the use of a special digital chip. This development may extend the fitting range of the ITE up to 85 or 90 dB HL. Above 90 dB HL, behind-the-ear (BTE), or, in a few cases, body aids are the better choice.

Factor 2. Clients may prefer in-the-canal (ITC) hearing aids. ITC hearing aids fit into the ear canal without extending very far out into the concha. They are less visible than full concha ITEs. This feature most often appeals to the client. However, ITC hearing aids are very small, their use is limited to milder hearing losses, and they accommodate fewer optional controls. For the elderly with limited manual dexterity or feeling in their fingertips, insertion, removal, and adjustment often are difficult because of the smaller size of the ITC aids.

Factor 3. Clients may need features that are available only with BTE or body hearing aids. BTE hearing aids may be ordered with contacts to connect auxiliary inputs that are necessary or desirable. Ears canals may be too small, soft, or deformed to accommodate an ITE. It is imperative to consider the client's need for special features when selecting the hearing aid type.

Problem 13-2. Selecting binaural versus monaural fitting.

Solution 13-2. Select binaural fitting unless otherwise indicated.

Procedure for Selecting Binaural Fitting

The major complaint of the potential hearing aid user often is inability to hear in background noise. With a monaural fitting his or her ability to discriminate speech in noise often is worse than without the monaural amplification, and the hearing aid ends up in a dresser drawer. In the long-term, it may be better for the clinician not to fit monaurally when the client's predominant complaint is difficulty hearing in noise, but, instead, to wait until the client can afford binaural hearing aids. For clients who can benefit from a monaural fitting in other listening situations, careful counseling concerning their expectations for hearing in noise is necessary.

Step 1. Determine that there is a pure-tone hearing loss in both ears. If so, the client may be a candidate for amplification.

Step 2. Determine that the two ears can be balanced to within 5 dB with amplification. If so, the client may be a candidate for binaural amplification.

Step 3. Determine that the two ears compliment rather than interfere with one another.
- Equalize the sensation levels between ears as nearly as possible.
- Administer a speech discrimination test binuarally.
- Compare the client's binaural speech discrimination scores with the results obtained previously in the monaural conditions. Binaural results that are as good or better than the better ear's monaural score indicate binaural compatibility.

Complicating Factors
Binaural fitting is contraindicated when:

Factor 1. One ear is normal (only one hearing aid is needed).

Factor 2. The two ears differ so greatly that they cannot be balanced with amplification.

Factor 3. Aiding both ears reduces the client's receptive communicative ability over aiding either ear alone.

Factor 4. If the client is in a limited listening environment that does not require listening when a competing message or noise is present.

Factor 5. The client can only afford one hearing aid and will obtain significant benefit from it.

Problem 13-3. Selecting the appropriate amplifier type.

Solution 13-3. Select the K-Amp unless otherwise indicated. The K-Amp hearing aid features a Class D, high-fidelity amplifier with its energy peak at 3000 Hz and an automatic volume control.

Complicating Factors
The K-Amp hearing aid may not be appropriate for some hearing losses.

Factor 1. Clients whose hearing losses exceed 65 dB HL may need greater amplification than the K-Amp can provide.

Factor 2. Experienced hearing aid users with hearing losses better than 65 dB HL who do not have complaints related to loudness tolerance problems may feel the amplification offered by the K-Amp is inadequate. For many of these individuals, the S-Amp provides an acceptable alternative to the K-Amp. The S-Amp, like the K-Amp, features a Class D, high-fidelity amplifier with its energy peak at 3000 Hz and an automatic volume control. However, it is a more powerful instrument.

Problem 13-4. Selecting the appropriate gain and frequency response.

Solution 13-4. Apply a formula to determine the 2-cc full-on gain by frequency response.

Procedure to Determine the 2-cc Full-On Gain by Frequency Response

The following steps are an adaptation on the Prescription of Gain/Output (POGO) formula (McCandless & Lyregaard, 1983). This formula was chosen for illustration because it is calculated in a straightforward and uncomplicated manner. If your supervisor prefers another formula, the multipliers in step 2, the correction factors in step 3, and the reserve gain in step 4 can be altered accordingly. Most real-ear systems allow you to choose among several formulas and then compute the desired gain automatically. When operating the real-ear system, the more complex and preferred Revised National Acoustics Laboratory (NAL) formula (Bryne & Dillon, 1986) can be chosen because the computer handles its complexity with ease. Whatever formula is used and regardless of how much computation the computerized real-ear system will complete for you, the following steps are necessary to determine the gain needed in a hearing aid. Gain must be determined separately for each ear.

Step 1. Determine the pure-tone air-conduction thresholds for the frequencies of 250, 500, 1000, 1500, 2000, 3000, 4000, and 6000 Hz in dB HL.

Step 2. Multiply each threshold obtained in step 1 by 0.5.

Step 3. Add the **insertion loss,** the ear canal resonance loss from the hearing aid or earmold in the ear canal, to the value obtained in step 2. If you can measure the ear canal response with a probe microphone, so much the better. Ear canal resonance varies greatly and, when changed, affects perceptions of hearing aid quality. When ear canal resonance cannot be measured directly, it may be grossly estimated from laboratory data as follows:

Frequency	Value
500	0.0
1000	0.0
2000	12.0
3000	17.0
4000	14.0

Step 4. Subtract 10 dB at 250 Hz and 5 dB at 500 Hz.

Step 5. Add 10 dB of reserve gain. **The resulting total is the 2-cc full-on gain desired.**

Complicating Factors

The hearing aid manufacturer does not build a hearing aid precisely to your specifications. Manufacturers choose a matrix from their stock that most closely approximates your order. Some of the digitally programmable hearing aids have a greater variety of gain-by-frequency choices that enable greater precision in filling your prescription. Unless you communicate clearly to the manufacturer who accepts your method of ordering, your order may not be filled correctly. This may cause delays in providing an appropriate fitting to your client. You should provide threshold, ear canal resonance and uncomfortable loudness (UCL) data to the manufacturer and determine the appropriateness of the hearing aid supplied to your client after it is received.

Problem 13-5. Selecting the appropriate maximum power output (MPO).

Solution 13-5. Limit the power output so that it does not exceed the client's UCL.

Procedure for Determining the Peak MPO

Step 1. Determine the pure-tone air-conduction UCLs for the frequencies of 500, 1000, 2000, and 3000 Hz in dB HL

Step 2. Add the **insertion loss** to the value obtained in step 1. See the values listed in step 3 of problem 13-4.

Step 3. Average the values obtained in step 2.

Step 4. Convert the average value obtained in step 3 to 2-cc coupler values by adding 4 dB. **The resulting total is the peak SSPL=90 desired.** When ordering, MPO is usually specified as peak power out and is fairly frequency specific. See Appendix H for a form to aid in the computation of 2-cc full-on gain and MPO.

Complicating Factors
See problem 13-4.

Problem 13-6. Gain requirements exceed maximum power output allowed by uncomfortable loudness levels. In this situation the client is likely to experience loudness tolerance problems.

Solution 13-6. Select an automatic volume control option. Rather than limit the maximum power output, and thereby the gain of the hearing aid for low intensity sounds, limit the gain for high intensity signals with an appropriate form of automatic volume control.

Problem 13-7. The client has good low-frequency hearing. With good low-frequency hearing the client may experience too much amplification in the low frequencies even with maximum low-cut filtering. The client's voice may sound "hollow," an experience akin to talking in a barrel. Worse yet, low frequency amplification may reduce discrimination in the higher frequencies by a spread of masking effect.

Solution 13-7. Select a low-cut trimmer option and vent the earmold on the BTE fitting or the case on the ITE fitting. The low-cut trimmer option reduces low-frequency amplification. Also, low-frequency energy escapes from vents. The larger the vent, the greater the amount of low-frequency energy escapes through it. Variable vents allow vent size to be changed to meet client needs without having to drill or fill single-sized factory-drilled vents. These two options give the clinician important control over troublesome low-frequency amplification.

Problem 13-8. Adjustment flexibility. Hearing aid fitting is closer to an exact science than it has ever been. However, some clients' needs may require periodic changes in frequency response, power, and feedback reduction. For such clients, an aid with trim potentiometers (pots) that allow adjustment to meet the special needs after the aid is ordered is a wise choice.

Solution 13-8. Select gain, frequency, power, and feedback controls. Many BTE hearing aids come from the manufacturer with three to four trimmer controls. On most ITE aids, trim pots are options that must be ordered and added to the cost of the hearing aid.

Complicating Factors
When ordering ITE or ITC hearing aids, there may not be enough room to select more than one trim pot option. In that case, the low-cut filter for reducing low-frequency energy often gives the most adjustment flexibility.

Problem 13-9. Telephone use. With many low-gain ITE instruments, the telephone can be amplified satisfactorily through the hearing aid and feedback prevented by holding the receiver a couple of inches away from the ear. Moderate and higher gain hearing aids are seldom usable directly with the telephone receiver without producing annoying levels of feedback. Few people prefer to remove a hearing aid and use a telephone amplifier. Therefore, with moderate and higher gain hearing aids, telephone use requires special accommodations.

Solution 13-9. Select a telecoil. A telecoil is a device that transduces the magnetic leakage from the telephone into an electrical signal that is amplified and transduced back into speech through the hearing aid. For most instruments, when the telecoil switch is on, the microphone is switched off, avoiding feedback when using the telephone with the hearing aid. Often the telecoil works better when the volume of the hearing aid is increased.

Problem 13-10. The client has a dead ear. Without hearing on one side of the head, an individual would be at a disadvantage in a situation in which another person was speaking softly on that side. Such a situation might occur in church, the theater, and like environments.

Solution 13-10. Select a contralateral routing of signal (CROS) fitting. The CROS fitting places a microphone encased in a BTE hearing aid on the unaidable ear and, through a wire around the back of the head, routes the signal to the good ear. Thus, a softly spoken signal on the dead side is heard. The wearer of the CROS fitting is still a monaural listener. All signals go into the same ear. A CROS fitting does not aid in localization or in selective listening in noise to any appreciable degree.

Problem 13-11. The client has a severe-to-profound sloping sensory or neural hearing loss requiring powerful amplification but has experienced

intolerable feedback problems with standard BTE fittings. The higher the level of gain required, the greater the possibility of feedback. Even with the newer feedback-reducing circuitry, hearing losses above 90 dB HL require such high levels of gain that feedback occurs. The answer is to increase the distance between the microphone and the speaker of the hearing aid and to place a barrier between them.

Solution 13-11. Select a Power CROS fitting. The power CROS fitting occludes the ear, separates the microphone from the speaker, and places a substantial barrier between the two.

Problem 13-12. The client wants to protect his or her investment. Clients with impaired function from stroke and other neurological conditions may be prone to losing hearing aids. Small children are more likely to break or lose their hearing aids than adults or older children. The hearing aid represents a significant financial investment to many users and may not be replaced if lost or damaged, unless insured.

Solution 13-12. Recommend the purchase of an extended warranty. Most hearing aid companies offer a variety of extended warranty plans that cover damage or one-time loss for a specified period of years. The aids may be insured as well, although insurance is a highly individualized decision. For most clients, it is best to present the options and allow the person plenty of time to talk over his or her individual needs with the family before deciding what is best for them.

Once a client is determined to be a candidate for amplification, a good earmold impression is essential. Earmold manufacturers provide step-by-step procedures for obtaining, judging the quality of, packaging for shipment, and ordering earmold impressions. However, some problems that may be encountered are not covered in readily available sources.

Problem 13-13. The client has excessively flaccid ear canals that expand disproportionately, creating earmold impressions that are too large. Earmolds made from such impressions create pressure and discomfort for the client.

Solution 13-13. Avoid overexpanding the ear canal when making the impression.

Procedure for Avoiding Overexpansion of the Ear Canal

Step 1. Withdraw the applicator at a slightly more rapid rate than usual when inserting the impression material.

Step 2. Use very slight pressure to smooth the impression material. Do not pack the impression material into the ear canal.

Problem 13-14. The client has a stiffer than typical cartilaginous ear canal with a great deal of jaw mobility visible in the ear canal. This condition may result in loose fitting earmolds or ITE aids and feedback.

Solution 13-14. Take an impression that will result in a tight-fitting earmold with a canal portion extending to the bony portion of the ear canal.

Procedure for Obtaining a Tight-Fitting Earmold with a Long Canal

Step 1. Place the impression block beyond the second bend of the ear canal to obtain a longer ear canal with the impression.

Step 2. Withdraw the applicator at a slower rate than usual when inserting the impression material.

Step 3. With your thumb, gently pack the impression material into the ear canal.

Step 4. After a minute or so of curing time, have the client rotate his lower jaw.

Complicating Factors

When their ear canals are touched, some individuals produce a **reflexive cough.** An earmold with a deep canal insertion may cause the client to feel a need to clear his or her throat and to lose voice after wearing the hearing aid. This is a case where a voice disorder may be induced by the earmold. When this happens, the earmold must be adjusted, and, perhaps, another type of hearing aid considered.

Problem 13-15. The ear canal is excessively hairy. It may be difficult to get a good impression, and removal of the impression material may pull the hair and cause the client discomfort.

Solution 13-15. Trim the hair.

Procedure for Trimming Ear Canal Hair

Step 1. Inform the client that to obtain a good impression of his or her ear canal some hair should be removed. Explain that the hair is only in the outer portion of the ear canal and that you can use small, blunt-tipped scissors to trim it. Obtain the client's permission to proceed.

Step 2. Place a towel on the client's shoulder to protect his or her clothing.

Step 3. Light the area of the ear canal well.

Step 4. Use one hand to straighten the ear canal and to stabilize the client's head.

Step 5. Cut the hair.
- Use small blunt-tipped scissors.
- Clip hair in small amounts beginning with those closest to the outside and proceeding inward. You must be able to see the tips of your scissors at all times.
- Clip the hair close to the canal wall, being careful not to cut the canal wall skin.

Step 6. Re-examine the ear canal.
- Determine whether the hair has been sufficiently removed. If not, repeat steps 5 and 6 until you are satisfied.
- Expect redding of the ear canal. Determine that there has been no injury to the ear canal wall. Injury to the ear canal wall precludes making an earmold impression until it is healed.

Bleeding is rare, but, if it occurs, small amounts of blood may be absorbed with a cotton swab. Excessive bleeding requires referral to a physician.

Complicating Factors
Removal of ear canal hair may be a relatively simple process or it may be more involved.

Factor 1. Difficulty of removal. When more than small amounts of wax are present, it adheres to the canal wall or combines with hair to provide a very strong barrier resistant to removal, and the process of hair removal becomes more involved and requires special instrumentation.

Factor 2. Supervisor preference. Even though ear canal hair removal is within the scope of practice of audiologists, some audiologists prefer not to clip ear canal hair. These factors complicate removal of excessive ear canal hair by introducing an extra step in the procedure, **referral to a medical specialist.**

Problem 13-16. Ear canal contains excessive cerumen.

Solution 13-16. Remove the cerumen. See Problem 12-1 in Chapter 12 for the step-by-step procedures for cerumen removal.

Problem 13-17. The ear canal appears abnormal. Ear canals may be infected with bacteria or fungus, contain soft tissue growths, have boils or pimples, be lacerated, or generally edematous.

Solution 13-17. Postpone making the earmold impression until after treatment by a physician, preferably one specializing in diseases of the ear. See the procedure for medical referral outlined in Chapter 12. Once appropriate amplification is selected, an earmold impression is made and ordered, the device(s) received, and the hearing aid orientation and follow-up are initiated.

Problem 13-18. What is the initial level of the volume control for a hearing aid placed on the patient for the first time?

Solution 13-18. Set the volume control to the user's most comfortable listening level, one third to two thirds of full-on volume.

Procedure for Setting User Level Volume

New users of hearing aids should not be left alone to set the volume control(s) of their hearing aids. Most binaural hearing aid users have difficulty balancing the gain to equalize the reception at the two ears. Also, many new users have forgotten the din of noise available to the normally hearing listener and set the volume control very low.

Achieving Initial Volume Control Setting

Real-ear evaluation enables you to approximate the gain setting of the hearing aid in the client's ear to a formula-generated curve and, thereby, achieve a gain control setting appropriate for the client's use. When real-ear evaluation is used with each aid in a binaural fitting, binaural balance is achieved. Monaural volume control adjustment and binaural balance may be achieved without real-ear measurement using the following steps:

Achieving Monaural Volume Control Adjustment

Step 1. Place one hearing aid in the client's ear and turn the volume control to approximately one half on.

Step 2. Ask from which ear the client hears. The client should report hearing from the amplified ear. If not, increase the volume.

Step 3. Ask the client if the sound could be louder. Be sure to use a quiet voice, or 30 dB HL through the audiometer in a sound field.

Step 4. Vary the volume control up and down between one third and two thirds on until the patient reports speech to be clear and the loudness comfortable.

Step 5. Do not fall into the trap of adjusting the volume control below one third on. If the client complains that the volume is too loud, reassure him or her that it will be adjusted later.

Achieving Binaural Balance

Step 1. After following steps 1-5 for Achieving Monaural Volume Control Adjustment, turn the hearing aid off, but leave it in the ear.

Step 2. Place the second hearing aid in the other ear and repeat steps 1-5 for Achieving Monaural Volume Control Adjustment, but leave the hearing aid on when finished.

Step 3. With the second aid adjusted and on, turn on the first aid.

Step 4. Ask whether the client hears in one ear, the other, or if the sound seems equal in both. Often, the client is unable to tell.

Step 5. Instruct the client that you are going to balance the hearing aids so that they are of equal loudness.

Step 6. Turn off one aid and ask the client to remember how loud the other sounds.

Step 7. Turn off the second aid and turn the first aid on. Ask the client if the second aid is softer, louder, or equal in loudness to the first aid.

Step 8. Repeat the comparison between the loudness of the aids, adjusting the volume control setting of the second aid until the client judges the aids to be equal in loudness.

Step 9. If the client complains that the hearing aids are too loud, turn the aids down toward one third gain until the client reports the loudness is comfortable. Repeat the balancing procedure.

Complicating Factor

Many clients who have experienced a gradual reduction in their hearing over several years, have difficulty accepting sound amplified to more normal hearing levels. Initial volume control settings may have to be adjusted to lower than desirable levels and wearing time for the aids limited so that the client can adjust to amplification gradually. It is best for clients to put on the hearing aids at an appropriate gain setting when they get up in the morning, to wear them all day, and to take them off when retiring for the evening. However, patience and several follow-up visits may be required for clients to make the adjustment to an appropriate gain setting.

Problem 13-19. The client is unfamiliar with the hearing aid(s).

Solution 13-19. Orient the client to the hearing aid(s).

Procedure for Hearing Aid Orientation

Step 1. Show the hearing aid(s) to the client. Identify the following:
• The microphone
• The volume control
• The battery compartment
• The vent

Step 2. If there are two hearing aids, show the client how to tell the left from the right. Most manufacturers color code ITE hearing aids; the right with a red dot and the left with a blue dot.

Step 3. Instruct the client on the insertion and removal of the ITE hearing aids or the BTE hearing aids and the earmolds.

Step 4. Have the client practice inserting and removing the hearing aids until he or she can successfully insert and remove the devices four times in succession.

Step 5. Identify the proper battery size and type, the battery life expectancy, and instruct the client in battery insertion and removal. Appendix I contains a battery life expectancy chart.

Step 6. Have the client practice the insertion and removal of the battery in the hearing aid until he or she can do it easily and without fear of breaking the battery drawer.

Step 7. Demonstrate acoustic feedback and explain its causes. Acoustic feedback usually will occur by turning the hearing aid to full volume and cupping it in your hand.

Step 8. With the hearing aid(s) turned off, have the client insert the aid(s) and adjust the volume control to a comfortable level. Talk to the client at a normal conversational level as he or she makes the adjustments.

Step 9. Observe the volume control position(s) when the client has achieved a comfortable setting. The control should be between one third and two thirds of full volume. Identify the volume control setting landmarks to the client.

Step 10. In binaural fittings, check to see that hearing is balanced. Preliminary balancing may be accomplished by snapping your fingers alternately on the right and the left side of the client's head. Care should be taken to produce the finger snaps at equal distances from the client's head. If the client has difficulty balancing the loudness of the hearing aids, see problem 13-16 for a procedure that can be used to balance binaural hearing aids.

Step 11. Explain and demonstrate the care and the maintenance of the hearing aids.
- Demonstrate how to clean wax from the receiver port with the wax loop.
- Demonstrate how to clean wax and dirt from the surface of the earmold or hearing aid case with a small soft brush.
- Explain that the hearing aid should be laid on a soft cloth with the battery removed when the client retires for the evening. Removing the battery at bedtime extends its life. Leaving the hearing aid exposed to the air overnight allows accumulated moisture to evaporate.

- Explain that the hearing aid should *not* be worn when swimming, in the spa, in the bathtub, or in the shower. It is an electronic device that can be damaged by water.
- Caution the client against exposing the hearing aid to excessive heat. The plastic case can deform or even melt if exposed to excessive heat. Care also should be exercised when using hair dryers.
- Caution the client against exposing the hearing aid to abrasive chemicals. It may be cleaned with a mild dishwashing soap and a damp cloth. The client should not use alcohol. The client should remove the hearing aid when using hair spray or getting a permanent.

Step 12. Instruct the client in the use of the telephone with the hearing aid.

Step 13. Practice use of the telephone with the hearing aid. The Time-of-Day Service may be dialed to provide a telephone signal for practice.

Step 14. Discuss realistic expectations for hearing aid use with the client.

Step 15. Discuss various listening situations.
- Identify situations in which a hearing aid will help and should be worn. For example, hearing aids should be worn when socializing with friends and family, watching television, and in other communicative situations.
- Identify situations in which a hearing aid will not help and should not be worn. For example, hearing aids should not be worn when operating loud equipment.
- Identify new and unfamiliar sounds for the client, for example, footsteps, keys, and birds singing.
- Discuss the effect of background noise on communication, especially in group listening situations.
- Discuss wind noise and the importance of changing position to avoid it, if possible.
- Discuss any changes in voice quality or volume perceived by the client.

Problem 13-20. The client experiences difficulty after leaving the clinic.

Solution 13-20. Contact the client at regular intervals to identify and deal with problems.

Problem 13-21. The client complains that the hearing aid is not working properly or feeds back.

Solution 13-21. Trouble-shoot the hearing aid and coupling system.

Procedure for Trouble-Shooting the Hearing Aid and Coupling System

Much of the following information for the performance check of the hearing aid was adapted from Niswander (1989). When a client presents with a malfunctioning hearing aid, at least four areas should be checked:

Power Supply

Step 1. Open the battery compartment and confirm that a battery is in place.

Step 2. Turn the hearing aid on in your cupped hand and listen for feedback. If feedback occurs, the aid is receiving power. Discontinue the power supply check. If no feedback occurs, continue the power supply check.

Step 3. Remove the battery and check the charge on the battery. If questionable or low, replace the battery with one from the client or the clinic's stock, if the client does not have one. Sometimes new batteries are low on power. Instruct the client to leave the seal on the zinc-air battery until ready to put it in the aid and not to reuse the tab.

Step 4. Note the position of the battery in the holder. If the battery is loose, the client may have used the wrong size replacement battery. Replace the client's battery with a proper size battery from the clinic's stock. Check for feedback. If feedback occurs, instruct your client regarding proper battery size. If no feedback occurs, continue the power supply check.

Step 5. Check to see that the battery is inserted properly, so that the positive (+) side is facing in the appropriate direction. Some batteries can be forced into the hearing aid upside down. The result is often a broken battery case hinge or battery case. If the battery is in backwards, remove the battery and reinsert it in its proper position. Check for feedback. If feedback occurs, shake the hearing aid gently back and forth. If the feedback becomes intermittent, tighten the case and replace the battery drawer, if needed. Check for feedback. If feedback occurs, the hearing aid is receiving power. Discontinue the power supply check. If no feedback occurs, discontinue the power supply check and return the hearing aid to the manufacturer for repair.

Mechanical Check

Check the integrity of the sound transmission channels, the hearing aid case, and the switches. Sound transmission channels include the earhook, tubing, and earmold on a BTE hearing aid. On an ITE aid, the sound transmission channels are the receiver tube and venting. On a body aid, sound transmission channels are the earmold, receiver, and cord.

Step 1. Check the integrity of the sound transmission channels.
- On BTE models, check the earhook and earmold tubing for loose connections and splits. These conditions may cause feedback above minimal settings and result in complaints of low volume. If loose or split earhooks or tubing are encountered, replace them.
- Sometimes, the power needs of the user are such that thick-walled tubing should be substituted for thin-walled tubing. Occlude the end of the earmold with your finger with the BTE hearing aid set at two thirds volume control. If feedback stops, the feedback problems experienced by the user are the result of improper coupling between the earmold and the client's ear. See "selecting a coupler system to prevent feedback" in the section on Coupler-system Check in this chapter. If feedback occurs, disconnect the tubing from the earhook and occlude the end of the earhook with your finger with the BTE aid set at two thirds volume control. If the feedback stops, the vent in the earmold is the cause of the feedback. Decrease the vent size until feedback stops. If the feedback continues, the tubing is the culprit. If the tubing is not loose or split, replace the thin-walled tubing with thick-walled tubing.
- On the BTE earmold or the ITE aid, check the receiver and vent holes. Sometimes they are blocked by earwax. If so, remove the earwax. Cup the ITE aid or the BTE aid attached to the earmold in your hand at full volume and listen for feedback. If the aid feeds back, reinstruct the client on the removal of earwax from the receiver and vent holes. Recommend a regular schedule of cerumen management to reduce the excessive accumulation of earwax in the ear canal.

Step 2. Check the integrity of the hearing aid case. The cases of the BTE or ITE aids may be cracked, or a thin area on an ITE may be worn through. A broken hearing aid case often results in feedback. A broken ITE case can cause physical damage to the concha or ear canal if insertion is attempted. Repair the case.

- If the hearing aid is under warranty, return it to the manufacturer for repair.
- If the hearing aid is not under warranty, and you have been trained to do so, repair the hearing aid. Otherwise, send the hearing aid to the manufacturer or other repair facility.

Step 3. Check the integrity of the switch(s).

- Attach the hearing aid to a hearing aid stethoscope.
- Turn the volume control rapidly up and down while listening to the hearing aid. Many volume control problems result not from a faulty switch, but from dirt or corrosion. If the volume is intermittent or crackles, spray a small amount of tuner cleaner on the control and work it vigorously up and down. When spraying the tuner cleaner, be sure to protect the microphone from the spray to prevent damage to it. If cleaning the volume control contacts does not eliminate noise and intermittency, send the hearing aid to the manufacturer for repair.
- Some hearing aids have an on-off switch, a telecoil switch, or a noise suppressor switch. Other hearing aids have some combination of these switches or none of them. Turn the on-off, telecoil, and noise-suppressor switches on and off while listening to the hearing aid through a hearing aid stethoscope. Note any popping sounds or intermittency. If either exists, use tuner cleaner and work the controls to clean. You should hear a change in sound quality when the noise suppressor switch is on. You should be able to tell when the on-off switch is working. You should use the telecoil switch with a telephone to determine whether it is working properly. If you have doubts that any switch is working properly, send the hearing aid for repair.

Performance Check

Step 1. Check the gain.

- Place the instrument, with the hearing aid on and the gain control set at minimum, in a hearing aid case with the cover open about 1½ inches.
- Increase the gain and note precisely where feedback starts.

• Estimate the gain by the amount of gain control rotation required for feedback to begin. Use the following volumes as guidelines.

Rotation	Gain Category
Last 1/3	Low gain ($<$ 45 dB)
Middle 1/3	Moderate gain (45-60 dB)
Initial 1/3	High gain ($>$ 60 dB)

Step 2. Check the MPO.
• Turn the instrument full-on and hold it 1-2 feet from your ear.
• Imagine that you are talking on the telephone and judge the interference level (loudness) of the feedback according to the following guidelines:

Loudness Judgment	MPO Category
Not too loud.	Low power ($<$ 110 SPL)
Would interfere.	Moderate power (110-125 SPL)
Very loud and shrill.	High power ($>$ 125 SPL)

Step 3. Check the frequency response.
• Attach a short (approximately 16 inch) stethoscope to the hearing aid.
• Set the gain to about one fourth rotation.
• Hold the hearing aid about 6 inches from your mouth and blow gently across the microphone. Judge the frequency response from the amplified sound according to the following:

Sound	Frequency Response
[ʃ] as in *she*	High-frequency emphasis
[ʃ] as in *shake*	Wide band
[ʃ] as in *shoe*	Low-frequency extended

Step 4. Check the frequency range.
• With the hearing aid attached to the short stethoscope and the gain set to one fourth rotation, say the following sounds into the instrument: [u] as in *Sue*, [ah] as in *father*, [i] as in *see*, [ʃ] as in *show*, and [s] as in *see*.
• Determine whether all the sounds are clearly amplified. Judge the frequency range on the clarity of the amplification as follows:

Sound	Frequency Range
[u]	$<$ 1000 Hz
[ah]	$<$ 1200 Hz
[i]	$<$ 3000 Hz
[ʃ]	2000 to 5000 Hz
[s]	4000 to 7000 Hz

Step 5. Check the signal-to-noise level.
- Attach a long (approximately 26 inch) stethoscope to the hearing aid.
- Set the gain to one half rotation.
- Hold the instrument at arm's length and bend the stethoscope tubing to achieve a soft listening level.
- Speak in a normal tone of voice and compare the level of speech signal to the noise level between the words and judge the signal-to-noise level as good or poor.

Step 6. Check the distortion.
- With the hearing aid attached to the long stethoscope and set at one half volume, speak into the hearing aid and note the clarity of the amplified speech.
- Judge the distortion as high or low.

Step 7. Check linear versus compression amplification.
- Attach a short stethoscope to the hearing aid.
- Adjust the gain to full on.
- Speak into the hearing aid in a normal voice at a close distance (approximately one half inch) and to one side of the microphone.
- Use a bend in the stethoscope to achieve a comfortable listening level.
- Judge whether speech becomes noticeably **distorted (linear)** or remains **unchanged (compression).**

Step 8. Check compression: input versus output.
- Place the instrument in a hearing aid case with the cover open about 1½ inches with the gain adjusted to full on.
- While listening to the feedback squeal, slowly decrease the gain of the instrument.
- Judge the signal as becoming gradually fainter (input compression) or remaining at the same level until just before feedback stops (output compression).

Coupler-System Check

The coupler-system consists of two parts. One part holds the hearing aid in the ear and the other part is the ear itself. The ITE case, the earmold and tubing of the BTE aid, and the snap-ring earmold of the body hearing aid are the parts that hold the hearing aid in the ear. Trouble-shooting these components was covered under the preceding section entitled Mechanical Check. Mention needs to be made of the interface between the earmold and the ear in two respects: the physical configuration of the pinna and ear canal and the power required by the hearing loss. If the ear canal appears highly mobile with swallowing, smiling, and talking and the hearing loss requires high gain, a Power CROS BTE may be the only fitting that will prevent unacceptable feedback.

Step 1.   Determine whether a tighter seal can be obtained by remaking the earmold or recasing the ITE.
   • If possible, remake the earmold impression following the procedure given in solution to Problem 13-14.
   • Order the earmold made of soft material or the ITE made with a soft canal.

Step 2.   If feedback remains a problem, recommend a Power CROS fitting.

After trouble-shooting the hearing aid power supply, mechanical aspects, and coupler system, the performance check may be skipped and a hearing aid analysis performed to determine its performance characteristics and to confirm that the aid is within electroacoustic specifications.

Problem 13-22. The electroacoustic performance of the hearing aid is not known.

Solution 13-22. Conduct an electroacoustic analysis of the hearing aid. Compare the hearing aid's performance to its specifications. After determining that the hearing aid is functioning properly, determine whether the hearing aid is appropriate for the individual's hearing loss.

Problem 13-23. The appropriateness of the hearing aid fitting for the client's existing hearing loss is not known.

Solution 13-23. Complete a hearing aid evaluation and selection procedure and compare the prescription derived with the hearing aid's performance.

**Procedure for Determining Appropriateness
of a Previously Fitted Hearing Aid**

The hearing aid evaluation involves obtaining the appropriate gain and MPO information based on the client's hearing loss. See the procedure for applying a formula to determine the 2-cc full-on gain by frequency response in Problem 13-4 in this chapter and the procedure for determining the peak MPO in Problem 13-5.

Problem 13-24. The hearing aid is not an appropriate fit for the client's hearing loss.

Solution 13-24. If possible, adjust the hearing aid so that it is appropriate for the client's hearing loss. If it is not possible to adjust the hearing aid, recommend the purchase of an appropriate hearing aid.

Procedure for Adjusting a Hearing Aid

The most effective method of adjusting a hearing aid is to follow the steps outlined below while, observing the results of the changes on real-ear measurements. However, without real-ear measurements, effective adjustments still can be made.

Step 1.   If one is available, adjust the trim pot controlling the frequency response to provide the most appropriate slope for the hearing loss as prescribed in the hearing aid evaluation.

Step 2.   Adjust the trim pot controlling the power of the hearing aid to within the MPO prescribed by the hearing aid evaluation.

Step 3.   Adjust the trim pot controlling automatic volume control to within the knee point prescribed by the hearing aid evaluation. **Compression knee point** is the signal intensity level where the amplification becomes less than linear. A compression knee point is presented graphically on hearing aid techical specification sheets an resembles a leg bent at the knee.

Step 4.   Vent the earmold or ITE case as necessary to reduce the hollow sound and the level of amplification of the client's own voice within the limits of feedback.

Step 5.   Adjust the feedback trim pot.
• Have the client turn the hearing aid volume control up until a comfortable listening level is reached.
• Trim the feedback trim pot to the point where the feedback disappears.

Complicating Factors
Several factors may complicate adjusting a client's hearing aid.

Factor 1. The client's hearing has changed significantly. Even a highly adjustable hearing aid may not be adjustable when the client's hearing has changed significantly. In that case, recommend a new hearing aid.

Factor 2. The hearing aid was fitted to the client less than a year ago. The hearing aid may have been inappropriate from the start and not be adjustable. You should take the hearing aid back and refund the client's money. A new hearing aid should be recommended.

Factor 3. The client was fitted inappropriately by someone else. The hearing aid may have been inappropriate from the start and be unadjustable. The dispenser of the hearing aid should take the hearing aid back and refund the client's money. A new hearing aid should be recommended. It is easier to admit and correct your own mistake than to point out someone else's mistake and ask him or her to correct it. The client should be encouraged to be tactful, but assertive. Communication with other professionals on the client's behalf should be cordial and free from accusation.

Assistive Listening Devices

In some situations, hearing aids provide limited benefit. In those situations, the client may be served better by an assistive listening device (ALD).

Problem 13-25. The client cannot function in low signal-to-noise ratios.

Solution 13-25A. Recommend a frequency modulated (FM) auditory training device. Several auditory training devices are available on the market. An FM system, as opposed to a hard-wire or induction loop system, is preferable. FM systems allow high sound quality, a high signal-to-noise ratio, and maximum mobility.

Solution 13-25B. Recommend an infrared system. These systems are commonly found in theaters, symphony halls, and public auditoriums. They also may be purchased by individuals. They depend on a light beam as a carrier signal and are limited to use in the same room. However, these systems provide an excellent quality signal and a high signal-to-noise ratio. In addition, they are significantly less expensive to purchase and operate than the typical FM auditory trainer.

Problem 13-26. The client's family complains that the television is too loud.

Solution 13-26A. Recommend an infrared personal listening system. This system can be adjusted by the individual to a comfortable listening level, while the rest of the family can listen to the television at more comfortable levels for them.

Solution 13-26B. Recommend an insert earphone hard-wired to the television. An alternative to the infrared personal listening system is the hard-wired insert earphone. The sound quality is usually good. However, when plugged into the television set, the internal speaker in the set is often disabled, precluding others from hearing the program. This option may be acceptable for an elderly adult living alone.

Problem 13-27. A client complains that his or her hearing aids do not improve conversation when riding in an automobile.

Solution 13-27A. A remote microphone. Hearing aids can be ordered with boot attachments for remote microphones. For individuals who spend a great deal of time communicating in an automobile, this solution may meet their needs.

Solution 13-27B. Turn the hearing aid next to the window off. For individuals who do not spend a great deal of time communicating in an automobile, it is less expensive to turn the hearing aid next to the window off than it is to purchase an additional hearing aid hard-wired to a remote microphone. Turning the hearing aid closest to the window off often reduces the competing noise enough that the hearing aid on the other side provides usable amplification.

Problem 13-28. A client has difficulty hearing a speaker in an auditorium, actors in a play, the sound track in a movie theater, or a live symphonic performance.

Solution 13-28. Recommend the use of an FM or infrared system. Even before the passage of the Americans with Disabilities Act (ADA) in 1992, many public gathering places provided amplification systems for the use of patrons with hearing-impairment. With the passage of ADA, more public meeting places provide these systems. Clients, however, may not be aware of the availability of assistive listening devices at theaters, churches, symphonies, and other public gatherings. It is a simple matter to inform clients and encourage them to use these devices.

Problem 13-29. A profoundly hearing-impaired person wishes to but is unable to use the telephone.

Solution 13-29. Recommend a telecommunication device (TTD). These devices allow messages to be typed and sent or received and displayed by those who have TDD units. Relay services are available so that the normal-hearing persons can communicate with hearing-impaired persons who have TTDs.

Problem 13-30. A profoundly hearing-impaired person wishes to but is unable to hear television programs.

Solution 13-30. Recommend a television captioning device. Television captioning devices produce printed dialogue along the bottom of the screen. More and more programs are closed-captioned and some television sets are now equipped with this option.

Problem 13-31. A profoundly hearing-impaired person cannot hear the telephone or doorbell ring.

Solution 13-31. Recommend a device that will convert the sound of the doorbell to a flashing light during waking hours and a vibration during sleeping hours. Flashing lights during waking hours and vibrations during sleep are effective signaling devices for individuals with hearing impairment. Signaling devices effectively keep persons with hearing impairment from becoming isolated. For elderly individuals who are hearing impaired and have life-threatening health conditions, it is especially important to be able to respond to signals from the outside world.

Problem 13-32. Deaf parents want to know when their baby awakens and cries during the night.

Solution 13-32. Recommend a device that converts the sound of the baby crying to light during waking hours and a vibration during sleeping hours. New parents, in particular, experience anxiety about the comfort and safety of their babies. For deaf parents, this anxiety may be increased because they cannot hear their baby's cries. Hearing parents hear their child cry and rush to provide for its needs. Deaf parents cannot respond to auditory signals, but can substitute voice-actuated lights or vibrators to inform them when their babies cry.

This chapter provided specific information in a problem-solving format covering issues related to managing hearing loss through amplification and assistive listening devices. The next chapter provides information related to managing hearing loss through modification of communicative behavior.

14

Audiologic Management Involving Modification of Communicative Behavior

Audiologic management for clients with hearing impairment includes training to enhance speech reception, speech production, and language production. Clinical methods designed to promote language production used in speech-language pathology are addressed in Hegde and Davis (1992) and are applicable to management of those problems in a client with impaired hearing. Management of disordered or delayed language in children often requires time intensive programs. Therefore, such management may be a part of education of the deaf programs. This chapter will concentrate on speech reception and speech production training for older children and adults. Techniques and materials used to modify communicative behavior vary depending on the age of the client, the age of onset of the hearing loss, the severity of the hearing loss, and the client's perceived need to improve his or her communication.

Speech Reception Management

The term speech reception management, also known as speech perception management, includes maximizing the client's skills in attend-

271

ing to speech that carries a primary message; repressing speech and other auditory signals that do not carry a primary message, and maximizing utilization of context to effect conceptual closure. Therefore, management techniques that emphasize synthesis of information should be used to enhance the receptive skills of the client who is hearing impaired. Analytic management techniques that concentrate on contrasting sounds should be restricted to establishing sound feature discrimination only when confusion between features exists and this confusion cannot be corrected by exercises that use information synthesis skills.

Most adults with acquired mild, moderate, and even severe hearing losses benefit from amplification to the point that there is little need for speech reception training. A few will need and seek additional help. However, adults with profound levels of hearing loss often need speech reception training to supplement auditory information provided through amplification. Adults and children who have received cochlear implants require training to make full use of the new auditory stimuli provided by the implant. Prelingually deafened children who are not cochlear implant candidates, or who receive limited cues to speech via amplification or tactile stimulation, should receive speech reception training integrated in a comprehensive language program.

Bisensory Training

Bisensory training emphasizes the integration of information between senses. For example, a person who is hearing impaired can get limited information from hearing and limited information from vision, but much more information from both than either sense alone. Two techniques that emphasize synthesis of information from the auditory and the visual systems are the Garstecki (1981) approach and the speech tracking approach (De Filippo & Scott, 1978; Mecklenburg, 1990). These approaches are suitable for use with adults and children 8 years of age or older with postlingually acquired hearing loss. These approaches will be presented in a problem-solving format.

Problem 14-1. The person with a hearing problem needs speech reception training.

Solution 14-1A. Utilize the Garstecki approach.

In the Garstecki approach, the goal is to increase the client's percent correct performance from baseline measures to previously stated levels after training. Therefore, a chart of behavioral change is helpful. Figure 14-1 presents such a chart. Figure 14-2 presents an explanation of the code used in Figure 14-1.

Procedure for Utilizing the Garstecki Approach in Speech Reception Training

Step 1. Establish and record a baseline. A **baseline,** the first measure of desired behavior, must be established and recorded. Baseline is chosen based on the client's expressed difficulties. For example, a client may report difficulty talking in a restaurant and a need to improve because his work requires frequent luncheon and dinner meetings. You may determine the client's baseline performance when unrelated sentences are the message (M_0), cafeteria/multispeaker babble (N-1) is the noise type, the signal-to-noise ratio is 0 dB (SN_0), and there are no background cues (C_0). The client will achieve a percent correct score which is then entered in the pretraining scores' column of the form in Figure 14-1 on the bottom row labeled *Baseline.*

Step 2. Next, present related sentences (M_1) to the client in the same noise type (N-1), at the same signal-to-noise ratio (SN_0), and with no cues (C_0). Enter the client's percent correct score for this condition on row 1, in the pretraining score column above the baseline. Message type is made more redundant while other factors are held constant and percent correct scores are obtained and recorded. If maximum performance is not obtained with the most redundant message type, then cues are varied until the most redundant cue level or maximum performance is reached. Next signal-to-noise ratio should be varied and the client's performance recorded. If necessary, noise type can be varied as well.

Step 3. Begin training. When the client's maximum performance has been obtained, then begin training at the level below maximum performance and move back to baseline. Training involves exercises similar to the ones used to obtain maximum performance. However, problems are discussed and practice at each level is continued until maximum performance at that level is reached. When the level of baseline is again reached and training completed,

Auditory-Visual Training Levels	Pretraining Score(s)	Posttraining Score(s)
11. M_3 N_0 SN_1 C_2	_____	_____
10. M_3 N_0 SN_1 C_1	_____	_____
9. M_2 N_0 SN_1 C_2	_____	_____
8. M_2 N_0 SN_1 C_1	_____	_____
7. M_1 N_0 SN_1 C_2	_____	_____
6. M_1 N_0 SN_1 C_1	_____	_____
5. M_0 N_0 SN_1 C_2	_____	_____
4. M_0 N_0 SN_1 C_1	_____	_____
3. M_3 N_0 SN_1 C_0	_____	_____
2. M_2 N_0 SN_1 C_0	_____	_____
1. M_1 N_0 SN_1 C_0	_____	_____
Baseline M_0 N_0 SN_1 C_0	_____	_____

Figure 14-1. A chart of behavioral change to be employed when utilizing the Garstecki approach. (Adapted from Auditory-visual training paradigm for hearing-impaired adults (p. 232) by D.C. Garstecki, 1981, *Journal of Rehabilitative Audiology, 14,* with permission.)

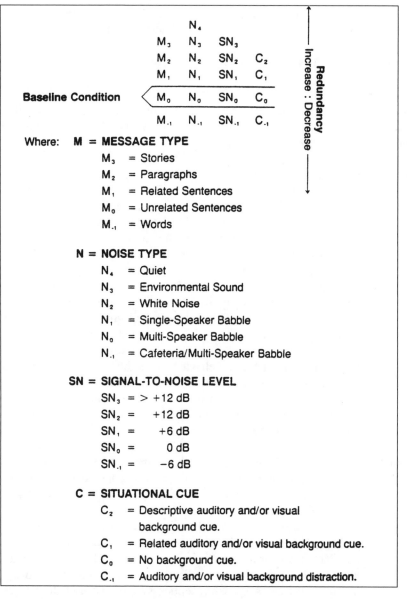

Where: **M** = **MESSAGE TYPE**
M_3 = Stories
M_2 = Paragraphs
M_1 = Related Sentences
M_0 = Unrelated Sentences
M_{-1} = Words

N = **NOISE TYPE**
N_4 = Quiet
N_3 = Environmental Sound
N_2 = White Noise
N_1 = Single-Speaker Babble
N_0 = Multi-Speaker Babble
N_{-1} = Cafeteria/Multi-Speaker Babble

SN = **SIGNAL-TO-NOISE LEVEL**
SN_3 = > +12 dB
SN_2 = +12 dB
SN_1 = +6 dB
SN_0 = 0 dB
SN_{-1} = −6 dB

C = **SITUATIONAL CUE**
C_2 = Descriptive auditory and/or visual background cue.
C_1 = Related auditory and/or visual background cue.
C_0 = No background cue.
C_{-1} = Auditory and/or visual background distraction.

Figure 14-2. A code for the symbols used on the chart of behavioral change to be employed when utilizing the Garstecki approach. (Adapted from Auditory-visual training paradigm for hearing-impaired adults [p. 230] by D.C. Garstecki, 1981, *Journal of Rehabilitative Audiology, 14,* with permission.)

differences in the percent correct score at baseline in the pre- and post-training columns will reflect the client's behavioral change.

Solution 14-1B. Utilize a speech tracking approach.

The speech tracking approach is scored in words per minute (WPM). In speech tracking, the clinician reads the stimulus material and the client repeats it verbatim utilizing both auditory and visual skills. One hundred percent correct performance is required.

Step 1. Establish a pretraining goal. This training is established by familiarizing the client with some of the stimulus materials and allowing the client to reference a copy, if necessary. The average time of three readings should be obtained. The goal of training is average time divided by the number of words in the reading materials. The materials may be a list of words, unrelated sentences, related sentences, a paragraph, or a story. Phrases for repetition should be limited to 2 to 10 words at a time during goal setting and training. Variables of message type, noise type, signal-to-noise ratio, situational cues, and group interaction may be used to simulate various listening situations in training.

Step 2. Establish a baseline of behavior. In addition to establishing a pretraining goal, it is necessary to establish a baseline of performance. The baseline of performance is the number of words per minute required for the client to repeat a pretraining passage at the beginning of the first session.

Step 3. Plot the client's progress. Obtaining the difference between the client's pretraining baseline score and his or her score for the last training passage for the session will enable the clinician to plot the client's progress.

There is some question whether the adults who were deafened prelingually can benefit from speech reception training. It is possible that neuronal patterns can be established for the individual whose primary communication mode is oral speech based on auditory cues. A speech reception system that uses the limited visual cues related to the formation of speech sounds or cues unrelated to speech sounds may not provide the oral language framework necessary to derive significant benefit from speech reception training. Thus, the adult who acquired language through sign language may not benefit from speech reception training.

However, an individual trained in cued speech may possess the oral language framework to benefit from speech reception training.

Unisensory Training

Unisensory training emphasizes the recognition of speech through one of three senses: hearing, vision, or touch. Both tactile and visual cues to speech are limited. Emphasis of auditory cues in unisensory training is called auditory training. Emphasis of visual cues in unisensory training is called speech reading. Utilization of tactile cues may result from tactile training. Visual cues are best learned in synthesis with auditory cues. Tactile cues can provide limited information about suprasegmental phonetic speech elements and are best learned in conjunction with visual cuing of auditory features.

Speech Production Management

Dynamic and context-sensitive elements in speech production tend to rely on auditory feedback for monitoring correct production. Repetitive patterned elements in speech production may be monitored more economically by tactile and proprioceptive sensory systems. Vocal pitch and vocal intensity levels are dynamic elements in speech production. Their patterns vary with communication situations. Timing and rhythm elements and articulatory processes vary more from the speaker's intent and less from varying external communication situations. For the latter features, once they are firmly established and practiced, tactile and proprioceptive feedback serve as cues for monitoring correct production. This division of labor within the sensory feedback mechanisms during speech production allows the speaker's auditory mechanism to be freed to monitor incoming messages from the environment and other speakers. Severe-to-profound hearing loss should not result in overall timing or articulatory speech production problems in postlingually, adventitiously deafened individuals. However, vocal pitch and intensity problems may be experienced. To produce speech, prelingually deafened children should learn to use feedback cues to timing, rhythm, vocal pitch, intensity level, and articulatory features.

To monitor vocal pitch and vocal intensity, hearing below 300 Hz and within the intensity range of the voice is necessary. Feedback regarding frequency from a tactile device is limited. However, for adventitiously deafened adults without adequate hearing in the range below 300 Hz, a tactile device may provide the feedback necessary to monitor vocal timing, rhythm, and intensity.

Articulation

A child who cannot not hear certain sounds in the language cannot imitate those sounds. Hence, the child cannot learn to produce them. Often the child does not even realize that he or she is missing a sound element. Cued speech identifies sound elements that are not visible with the use of supplemental hand positions and shapes. When the speech-language pathologist uses cued speech while working with a hearing-impaired child on speech production, cuing identifies sound elements that are not familiar to the child. The speech-language pathologist or rehabilitative audiologist can then train the child to approximate the speech sound and to associate the new sound with the cue for it. Cuing of connected discourse then may enable the hearing-impaired child to generalize the use of the newly acquire sound.

Language Management

Oral-Aural

The most appropriate language for a child to learn is the language of his or her culture. Early identification of hearing loss and teaching of language through the combination of auditory cues and cued speech will enable the child to acquire language of the primary culture.

Other language issues are presented by adults suffering from combined aphasia and hearing loss. Those issues are best managed through a team effort of the audiologist and speech-language pathologist.

Manual

Manual communication systems are appropriate for children who are not candidates for cochlear implants and do not respond to auditory information. With an overlaid language disorder, some hearing-impaired children respond to sign language as a means of acquiring language and communicating much more readily than to an auditory system. Manual communication is appropriate for these children. Such children should be referred to an educator of the deaf.

Problem 14-2. A person elects communicative management in lieu of or before obtaining a hearing aid.

Solution 14-2. Schedule the person for a 1-hour session.

Procedure for Demonstrating Client Benefit from Amplification

The goals of the session are to obtain baseline measures and to establish training goals (a) using vision and audition, (b) using audition alone without amplification, and (c) using audition with amplification. Amplification is provided by an auditory trainer.

Step 1. In implementing the following steps 1 through 6, use the Garstecki method outlined in Solution 14-1A. Obtain a baseline for the condition where the client uses both unaided audition and vision.

Step 2. Obtain a maximum performance level for the condition where the client uses both unaided audition and vision.

Step 3. Obtain a baseline for the condition where the client uses unaided audition only.

Step 4. Obtain a maximum performance level for the condition where the client uses unaided audition.

Step 5. Obtain a baseline for the condition where the client uses audition aided with an auditory trainer set to compensate for his or her hearing loss.

Step 6. Obtain a maximum performance level for the condition where the client uses audition aided with an auditory trainer set to compensate for his or her hearing loss.

Step 7. Compare the results of the three conditions. The client should score higher on the multisensory condition than on the auditory only condition and achieve maximum performance at a more difficult level than in the auditory only condition alone. The client should score higher and achieve maximum performance earlier in the aided auditory condition than the unaided auditory condition.

Step 8. Discuss the results with the client before beginning training. Ask the client to consider the following questions:
- What are the limitations of relying on vision and unaided audition alone?
- What are the limitations of relying on unaided audition alone?
- What are the advantages to aided audition?
- What are the disadvantages of unaided audition?

Do not draw a conclusion for the client. If the client concludes that he or she needs amplification, reinforce that conclusion and schedule the client for a hearing aid evaluation before proceeding to step 9. If the client has ordered a hearing aid and is waiting for its arrival, proceed to step 9 when the hearing aid is received. If the client is unable to use or rejects amplification, skip to step 12.

Step 9. Schedule the client for another session and establish baseline and maximum performance goals using vision and audition aided by the new hearing aid(s) and audition alone aided by the new hearing aid(s).

Step 10. Begin training in the auditory condition alone aided by the client's new hearing aid(s).

Step 11. When training is complete in the auditory condition alone, retest the condition where vision and audition, aided by the new hearing aid(s), are used. Significant improvement should be observed in the combined condition. If so, skip to step 15. If not, go to step 14.

Step 12. Train the client to criteria for audition alone without the auditory trainer.

Step 13. Train the client to criteria for visual and auditory cues together without the auditory trainer. If the client changes his or her mind regarding amplification at any time during this step, facilitate the acquisition of hearing aids and proceed to step 14. If the client has not acquired amplification and goals for speech reception training have been met, conclude training.

Step 14. Train the client to criteria for vision and audition aided by the new hearing aid(s).

Step 15. If the client has met current training goals, determine the need for additional training, schedule additional sessions to determine new goals, or end receptive communication training.

Problem 14-3. A person who has obtained one or more hearing aids continues to have difficulty with receptive communication.

Solution 14-3. Refer the person for receptive communication management.

Procedures for Referring a Client for Management of Speech Reception

Step 1. Inform the client of the need for further services in the form of receptive communication training.

Step 2. Schedule the client for a session to determine baseline performance levels and to develop goals.

Step 3. Obtain the client's agreement to enroll in a specific number of 1-hour weekly sessions. This may be for a semester or 6 weeks or more, based on the projected rate of client progress.

Problem 14-4. A person has been scheduled for receptive communication training. There are no baselines for receptive communicative behavior.

Solution 14-4. Establish baselines.

Procedure

For the Garstecki method, begin at M_0, N_0, SN_0, and C_0 and determine a percent correct score. For the speech tracking method, determine a word per minute rate utilizing Utley lip reading sentences, CID Everyday Sentences, or monosyllabic words.

Problem 14-5. A person has been scheduled for receptive communication training. There are no goals for receptive communication training.

Solution 14-5. Establish goals.

Procedure for Establishing Goals

Step 1. Discuss with the client what he or she hopes to achieve from receptive communication training. Set realistic goals. For example, a realistic goal would be to increase the baseline percent correct or word per minute score. An unrealist goal would be to score 100% correct on a post-training probe measure or to exceed more words per minute in speech tracking than is possible for this client and this clinician and with the material being used.

Step 2. Specify a criterion by which progress is measured. In the Garstecki method, training should increase the percent correct score at a particular level until no increase in percent correct score is obtained and post-training evaluation at that particular level matches the maximum correct score obtained at that level. In the speech tracking method, the client is required to repeat with 100% accuracy the materials the clinician presents. WPM is plotted for each trial until the client does not improve his WPM or until the averaged WPM score obtained with similar materials with which the client is familiar is reached.

Problem 14-6. A person has been scheduled for receptive communicative training. Training materials do not exist.

Solution 14-6. Develop training materials.

Procedure for Developing Training Materials

Step 1. Determine an appropriate level of materials according to the client's age, educational background, experience, and the degree of difficulty he or she experiences. Be sure to consider cultural differences.

Step 2. Examine existing materials and choose materials that can be adapted to your purposes.

Step 3. Adapt the materials or develop new materials appropriate for the client.

Step 4. Prepare several steps in the evaluation and training procedures in advance.

Step 5. Present your materials to a colleague, family member, or friend prior to using them with the client.

Step 6. Request comments from the person helping you regarding the appropriateness of the materials to the client and the training session goals.

Problem 14-7. A person has been scheduled for receptive communication training. When is it appropriate to conclude training?

Solution 14-7. When training criteria that indicate the client is not progressing or that goals have been achieved.

Procedure for Concluding Training

Step 1. Keep track of performance after every trial and chart behavior.

Step 2. Have criteria for performance clearly marked on the form and when criteria are achieved conclude training at that level. If criteria are not obtained or after five successive trials without an increase in the client's performance, conclude training at that level.

Problem 14-8. A person has been scheduled for receptive communication training. The client has no idea how he or she is expected to perform in this situation.

Solution 14-8. Compare the clinician's and the client's performance.

Procedure for Comparing the Clinician's and the Client's Performances

Assuming that the clinician has normal receptive communicative ability, his or her performance can be used as a measure of expectations for normal performance.

Step 1. Using a diagram of the client's aided hearing superimposed on an SII graph and a diagram of the clinician's hearing imposed on an SII graph, note the differences in percent correct scores. Establish that the client is not expected to perform better than the clinician.

Step 2. Have the client administer a parallel set of materials to the clinician.

Step 3. Compare the client's performance to the clinician's performance, taking into consideration the difference between the client's aided abilities and the clinician's hearing. Discuss appropriate expectations for the client in light of the comparison.

Problem 14-9. A person with disordered speech related to hearing impairment has been referred for speech production training. When to service the person and when to refer the person are not clear?

Solution 14-9. Refer the person if you are not trained or equipped to deliver the specific services needed.

Many audiologists are trained, equipped, and effective in providing speech production training with individuals who are hearing-impaired. Those clinicians may provide the services or refer to speech-language pathologists who are trained, equipped, and are effective in providing speech production training with clients who are hearing impaired.

Problem 14-10. A person with disordered speech related to hearing impairment has been referred for speech production training. The initial step is not clear.

Solution 14-10. Evaluate the client's speech skills.

Procedure for Evaluating Speech Skills

Step 1.   Evaluate the prosody of the individual's speech.

Step 2.   Evaluate vocal pitch level.

Step 3.   Evaluate vocal intensity level.

Step 4.   Evaluate articulation of the individual.

Problem 14-11. A person with disordered speech related to hearing impairment has been referred for speech production training. The training sequence is not known.

Solution 14-11. Rely on auditory, visual, and tactile cues to sound production to help the person produce sounds correctly. Design your management program based on distinctive feature analysis.

Problem 14-12. A person with disordered speech related to hearing impairment is in speech production training. When to conclude training is not clear.

Solution 14-12. Conclude training when criteria have been achieved.

Procedure

Plot a learning curve specifying percent correct productions by trial. If criteria are not obtained after five successive trials without an increase in the measure of behavior, conclude training at that level.

In Chapter 14 management of communicative behavior in the client with hearing impairment has been discussed and specific techniques put forward to manage specific problems. In the next chapter, management involving psychosocial issues will be addressed.

15

Audiologic Management Involving Psychosocial Variables

The client who seeks services from an audiologist because of hearing loss has more than a hearing problem. Often the client lacks information about his or her hearing loss, its causes, and the treatment options that are available. The audiologist can provide informational counseling. However, the client often suffers loss and needs an understanding and empathic listener. The audiologist can provide affective counseling. **Informational counseling** addresses clients' need to know. Its goal is to inform clients by the presentation of factual information. Sometimes factual information is all that clients need to effect positive behavioral change. **Affective counseling** addresses clients' emotions and attitudes that result from hearing loss. **Audiologic counseling** includes informational and affective counseling related to hearing loss and the adjustment to it.

In this chapter, psychosocial variables are defined to include vocational, educational, psychological, and social issues. The client may experience social and vocational problems associated with his or her hearing loss. The audiologist may be the professional who refers the client for social and vocational services and advocates for services for the client.

The parents of children with hearing impairment may find the educational alternatives available for their children bewildering. The audiologist can help parents sort out the issues and choose appropriate alternatives for their children. In addition, the audiologist may be in the best position to advocate for appropriate educational placement for the child.

Audiologic Counseling

Audiologic management may include counseling for clients' informational and affective needs related to hearing loss. Effective counseling requires training and practice. Some course work in communicative disorders includes techniques of informational counseling. Many training programs in communicative disorders offer courses that teach affective counseling techniques. Opportunities to practice counseling skills are made available to students through practicum experiences.

Effective counseling requires a working relationship between the client and the professional. Working relationships are based on a rapport between the client and the professional. **Rapport** implies that the client trusts the professional. With rapport, the client can work cooperatively with the professional.

Problem 15-1. Rapport has not been established between the client and the audiologist.

Solution 15-1. Establish rapport.

Establishing Rapport with Adults

This procedure is based on information presented by Roberts and Bouchard (1989). The steps that follow assume an initial meeting between you and the client. Initial meetings with clients by audiologists most often are followed by a hearing evaluation and this condition is assumed here. However, the procedure for establishing rapport may be adapted to fit situations other than meeting the client for the first time prior to hearing evaluation.

Step 1. Smile as you greet the client. Make sure that your right hand is free to shake hands. Be aware that institutional, regional, gender, and cultural rules of social interaction can determine whether hands are shaken and who initiates the handshake. For example, in some regions of the country and with some cultural groups, if the client is a man, the clinician should extend his or her hand. If the client is a woman, she should be allowed to initiate the handshake, if she desires to. One of the authors (BRK) provides audiology services for prison inmates. Institutional rules strictly prohibit touching prisoners, including the shaking of hands.

Step 2. Ask the client to come with you.

Step 3. Seat the client in the examination room or conference area and be seated at an angle across from them without any objects between you.

Step 4. Observe the client's posture, sitting position, and speech.
- Leaning back with arms folded across the chest and legs crossed may indicate a defensive posture. Be careful to take all possible meanings into consideration. Arms folded and legs crossed simply may indicate a full bladder.
- Leaning forward with hands on the knees and legs uncrossed may indicate receptiveness.
- A statement by the client that he or she is sure that whatever management the clinician suggests will not work indicates a lack of receptiveness on the part of the client.

Step 5. Determine whether the client's posture and speech indicates openness and trust. If it does, go to step 10. If it does not, go to step 6.

Step 6. Assume the client's posture as you begin the initial interview. Restate the client's verbal expressions.

Step 7. During the interview, as the client changes position, subtly change your position accordingly. Continue to restate the client's statements.

Step 8. After following the client's lead for a few minutes, lead by changing positions and observing the client's response. You also may lead verbally using techniques of confrontation, verbal reframing, and suggesting to the client that he or she has the ability and potential to set goals and achieve results. Your lead has been established when the client adjusts his or her posture to closely match yours and his or her speech toward setting appropriate goals.

Step 9. Shape the client's posture and sitting position to a relaxed and open one. The assumption is that posture and body position reflect the person's emotional and relational states and that, by changing the posture and body position, you affect those states. Shape the client's attitudes as reflected by their speech to setting-specific behavioral goals. An excellent discussion on establishing counseling goals in audiologic management is found in Roberts and Bryant (1992).

Step 10. With a smile and a friendly manner, gather oral case history information with informal questioning. For example, you might begin with the question, "What brought you here today?"

Step 11. After the initial interview, inform the client that you are going to evaluate his or her hearing.

Step 12. During the evaluation, ask the client frequently if he or she understands or has any questions. By the end of the evaluation, rapport should be firmly established. Rapport is essential for effective long-term counseling relationships. However, it is desirable, but not necessary, in many clinical contexts. For example, effective diagnostic evaluation may be accomplished without rapport.

Procedure with a Young Child

Step 1. Greet the parent(s) and ask the parent(s) to bring the child and come with you.

Step 2. When greeting the child initially, position yourself so that you are on the same plane as the child, smile, and say "Hello, (the child's name)."

Step 3. Establish rapport with the parent(s). See Problem 15-1

Step 4. While gathering information from the parent(s), ask the child questions as found appropriate. For example, the parent(s) may mention that the child has allergies. You may ask the child, "Do you have a pet?" and "What is your pet's name?" By asking the child questions in a friendly and nonthreatening manner, he or she is included in the interview process. Also, the basis for relationship between you and the child is begun in the safety of his or her parents' presence.

Step 5. Offer the child your hand. If the child takes your hand, lead him or her to the examination area. If the child hesitates and looks toward the parent, go to step 6. If the child proceeds with you without checking with the parent, rapport has been established.

Step 6. Ask the parent to accompany you to the examination area.

Step 7. In the examination area, inform the child about the evaluation procedure.
- Position yourself on eye level with the child.
- Use age-appropriate language.
- Demonstrate the signals the child will hear.
- Demonstrate the response the child will give.
- Do not use the word "test."
- Gently stroke the child's hand or arm while talking to him or her. Touch can often establish rapport. However, it can break rapport. Be observant. Some children do not like to be touched and will withdraw. If physical withdrawal from your touch occurs, cease and desist. More time relating to the child may be necessary to gain rapport to obtain the child's cooperation with whatever procedure you wish to initiate.

Step 8. Place the earphones on the child. If the child allows the earphones to be placed, trust is established. Commence testing. If the child rejects the earphones, more time must be taken to establish trust. If more than a single session is required, reschedule the child for a second appointment. Once rapport has been established, you are in a better position to determine the client's understanding and the emotional effects of his or her hearing loss.

Problem 15-2. The client does not understand his or her hearing loss and its effect on him or her.

Solution 15-2. Inform the client how the hearing mechanism is structured and how it functions.

Procedure for Informational Counseling About Hearing Loss

Step 1. Encourage the client to ask questions as they arise.

Step 2. Give a brief overview of the anatomy and physiology of the auditory system. Utilize a color chart of the ear. The chart should be large enough to reveal the detail to which you refer. Frontal sections of the temporal area in color are available from several sources.

Step 3. Give a brief overview of types of hearing loss.

Step 4. Identify the client's hearing problem by type and give specific examples of situations where the client may experience difficulty communicating.

Step 5. Ask the client to describe situations in which he or she experiences difficulty communicating.

Step 6. Ask the client to relate his or her hearing loss to the communication difficulty described.

Problem 15-3. A client has seen an otologist who diagnosed hearing loss and recommended surgical treatment. The client has come to you for information regarding management options available in lieu of surgery.

Solution 15-3. Schedule the client for an informational counseling session.

Procedure for Conducting Informational Counseling about Management Options

Step 1. If available, obtain a report from the treating physician.
  • Review the report and determine the diagnosis and recommended treatment.
  • Determine all management options appropriate to the clients specific condition.

Step 2. Give the client an overview of the diagnosed condition and how the surgical treatment is designed to work.

Step 3. Present all management options appropriate for the client's specific condition. When the cause of the hearing loss is not active pathology or there is no treatment to arrest the progression of

the hearing loss, as in otosclerosis, medical treatment may be designed to restore hearing. An alternative management option to partial restoration of hearing without surgery is amplification.

Step 4. Encourage the client to ask all the questions he or she has. Answer them appropriately.

Step 5. Encourage the client to express concerns or apprehension. Acknowledge them.

Step 6. Encourage the client to evaluate and select an appropriate management option.

Step 7. Reassure the client that the management option he or she has chosen is appropriate.

Problem 15-4. The emotional effects of identification of hearing loss on the client are unknown. How do I probe the understanding and emotional effects of the hearing loss upon the client?

Solution 15-4. Ask the client.

Procedure for Probing for Emotional Effects of Hearing Loss

Step 1. Establish rapport with the client before testing.

Step 2. Be direct, but gentle, as you inform the person of his or her hearing loss. For example, "Mrs. Jones, as you suspected, you have some hearing loss."

Step 3. Ask the client how he or she *feels* about having hearing loss? For example, "How are you feeling?"

Step 4. Wait for the client to answer. Be patient and attentive. When dealing with loss, clients often must feel before they can process information. Look for signs of emotion, such as tearing. Allow the client to speak first. Most people feel uncomfortable with long silent spaces and eventually will speak to fill them. It is not as important for clients to share their feelings as it is that you ask them to and give them an opportunity to share.

Problem 15-5. The client is having difficulty dealing with the hearing loss.

Solution 15-5. Provide affective counseling.

Procedures for Affective Counseling

Styles in affective counseling are as diverse as the problems and the people involved. Several general principles are involved:

- When in doubt ask questions. For example, "How are you feeling?" If the client acknowledges some feeling, ask him or her to tell you what thoughts are associated with times when he or she feels the feeling named, until you have the individual talking about his or her feelings. Once they are talked about, feelings are often better understood and dealt with.
- Do not offer solutions to feelings. Respond with questions that help the individual to identify the problem and to initiate his or her own solution to the problem. Be a sounding board for the client.
- When the client is ready and initiates the process, help the client to identify alternative approaches to problem solving and guide him or her in choosing an appropriate alternative behavior by reinforcing conclusions that will have a positive impact on solving the problem.

Problem 15-6. The client's response criterion is too conservative or too liberal. Some clients guess less at what they hear than is appropriate for them to communicate effectively. Others compensate for their inability to hear by guessing more than they should. An effective response criterion enables the individual with impaired hearing to have confidence in what he or she hears, to guess appropriately when he or she has not heard clearly, and to ask for repetition when the message was not heard clearly and guessing is not appropriate.

Solution 15-6. Modify the client's response criterion.

Procedure to Modify Client's Response Criterion

In the chapter on diagnostic strategy, same-different nonsense syllable testing and β scoring were introduced to measure the client's response criterion. Recall that β, a measure of response criterion, results from the client's knowledge of context of the message and the relative costs and gains he or she associates with responding. Beta scores of 1.0 are statistically ideal responses. Listeners with normal hearing tend to score at 1.0 on the same-different nonsense materials. Beta scores greater than 1.0 indicate a criterion that is more conservative than the statistical ideal, whereas β scores less than 1.0 indicate a criterion that is more liberal than the statistical ideal. When clients have low speech discrimination scores, relatively high d' scores and β scores other than 1.0, their response criterion is inappropriate and needs to be modified.

Whether a client's response criterion is too liberal or too conservative, the following steps should be instituted. The behaviors that are reinforced differ for liberal and conservative responders.

Step 1. Begin with paired-stimulus materials that are easily discriminated in a forced-choice paradigm. For example, the words *it* and *blackboard* are more easily discriminated than the words *it* and *hit.* A forced choice requires the client to identify the pair as different or as the same.

Step 2. Positively reinforce all responses for **the client whose criterion is too conservative.** For adults, positive reinforcement may be a comment, such as, "Good. You got that one correct!" or "That was a good guess!" Plot scores across trials with 5 points for each correct response and 0 points for each incorrect response. This is to convince the person with too conservative a criterion that guessing more will result in being right more often and that some error is tolerable. Positively reinforce only correct responses for **the client with too liberal a criterion.** For adults, offer comments such as, "Good. You got that one correct," when he or she responds correctly, and, "That is incorrect," when he or she misses one. Plot scores across trials with 1 point for each correct response and -1 point for each incorrect response. The object is to convince the person with too liberal a criterion that not being wrong is as important as being right.

Step 3. Increase the difficulty of the paired stimulus materials.

Step 4. Repeat step 2.

Step 5. Help the client generalize response criterion through structured group sessions.

Another situation where counseling is appropriate is when a client recognizes the need for but rejects amplification. A client who is unprepared, ill-informed, or unwilling to accept a hearing aid most likely will be a failure at hearing aid use and may be spoiled for hearing aid use later when he or she has even greater need. For such clients, an alternative to immediately obtaining a hearing aid may be counseling. The purpose of counseling this client is to have him or her verbalize, accept, and initiate goals to meet his or her communicative needs. Roberts and Bryant (1992) present specific techniques to accomplish this purpose.

Let us assume that a woman in her sixties has insisted that her husband is hard-of-hearing and scheduled an appointment for him. The husband insists that he hears well for his age but that people mumble a lot. He admits little perceived difficulty hearing except in noise which he assumes is a problem everyone faces. After his hearing test is completed, a sloping high-frequency hearing loss is identified. He listens to the audiologist's explanation of his hearing loss and its possible effect on his receptive communication and acknowledges that his hearing is not normal. He still may elect to wait until his problem is severe enough to warrant treatment. He has the option to terminate the relationship. The client has the ultimate right to decide the management strategy. However, in this example, the client needs help in accepting his hearing loss and an option that may help him communicate more effectively. To suggest, at this time, that he needs a hearing aid may very well cause him to abort the management process. He may go somewhere else for services in a year or two, but he probably will not come back to you. Therefore, the clinic has lost a client and the client has suffered longer than may have been necessary with communication difficulty.

Problem 15-7. The client is reluctant to accept amplification as a management option at this time.

Solution 15-7. Family-oriented counseling with a needs assessment focus.

Procedure for Family-Oriented Counseling with a Needs Assessment Focus

A recommendation is made for family-oriented counseling, the sole purpose of which is to clarify the issue that the client has a hearing loss and that the client feels there are no significant communication problems resulting from the hearing loss whereas his or her spouse feels that there are such problems. For a good overview of counseling techniques, see Meier and Davis (1993).

Step 1. Both client and spouse are asked to keep separate journals for the few days between this and the next appointment, noting specific instances in which he experiences communication difficulty. They are not to share their journals or to discuss what they have noted with each other.

Step 2.   The next appointment will be a counseling appointment, the focus of which is to review the notes of the husband and wife and to discuss what they indicate. In this session both the client and his wife should be asked: "What do you think about this situation? How did you feel in that situation?" The person's thoughts and feelings about each situation should be restated by the clinician and the other person.

Step 3.   If at this point the client's comments indicate an acceptance of communication problems, he and his wife can be informed regarding general rehabilitative options available to them and scheduled for a follow-up appointment. If the client still does not acknowledge communication difficulties, or the exercise of noting communication problems indicates little difficulty related to hearing loss, the client can be dismissed.

Step 4.   The client and his wife should be reassured that, should they wish to do more about the hearing loss, they are welcome to return for further services. Also, the client should be scheduled for annual hearing evaluation. Hearing seldom improves and often gets worse.

Problem 15-8. The client questions the need for two hearing aids.

Solution 15-8. Inform the client about the benefits of two hearing aids in establishing auditory figure-ground relationships.

Complicating Factors

Factor 1.   The client cannot afford two hearing aids at this time.

Factor 2.   The client can benefit from one hearing aid.

Factor 3.   Client preference is to try one before purchasing a second hearing aid.

Problem 15-9. The client has withdrawn from situations that give him or her difficulty.

Solution 15-9. Recommend assertiveness training.

Procedure for Assertiveness Training

Assertiveness training should have as its goal developing client behavior that recognizes communication problems and is appropriately proactive in solving them. Assertiveness training should never become aggressiveness training. Assertive behavior practiced appropriately should not offend others. Instead, the parties involved can mutually benefit from more effectively communicating their needs. Scores of techniques for teaching assertiveness are available in the popular and professional literature and are easily adapted for use in the clinic.

Step 1. Ask the client to identify three to five situations in which he or she experiences communication problems.

Step 2. Ask the client to rank the problems he or she identified in step 1 from least to most difficult.

Step 3. Beginning with the least difficult problem, ask the client to identify the context in which the difficulties arise and the other persons most often involved.

Step 4. Ask the client to identify three to five ways in which he or she could respond to the situations and the persons.

Step 5. Have the client examine the possible consequences of the different responses identified in step 4.

Step 6. Have the client choose a method of asserting his or her right to effective communication.

Step 7. Role play the method chosen in step 6 with the client.

Step 8. Assign the client to report on one instance in which he or she used the strategy practiced in the clinic on the outside. Praise the client's efforts, no matter how timid.

Step 9. Assign the client more instances where he or she uses the strategy in subsequent sessions until the client reports a mastery of the strategy for the least difficult of his or her communication situations.

Repeat steps 1 through 9 for other communication difficulties identified in order of increasing difficulty. The client should gain confidence in self assertion for effective communication and report feeling more confident in difficult communication situations. Management may be concluded at this time with periodic maintenance sessions scheduled.

Problem 15-10. The client extends the diagnostic or management session by visiting, not from a need for information or dealing with the effects of the hearing loss, but from loneliness.

Solution 15-10. Referral to outside services.

Problem 15-11. The client needs emotional, vocational, or educational support working through the effects of the hearing loss. How do I determine when to counsel the client and when to refer the client for professional counseling?

Solution 15-11. You should consult your supervisor before you make diagnostic statements or management decisions.

Procedure for Clearing Diagnostic Statements and Management Decisions

When considering referral out of the practicum setting for additional services, it is imperative that you discuss the situation with your supervisor. Your supervisor must make the final judgment. If your supervisor believes that the client's problems require professional expertise beyond your skill to deliver and his skill to supervise, referral should be made. If you have the skill to provide the service and your supervisor is willing to supervise counseling sessions, you may initiate counseling. Be aware that, after beginning counseling with a client whose problems are later revealed to require referral, the client can be referred at that time.

Problem 15-12. How do I refer clients to a professional counselor for psychological, emotional, or interpersonal counseling.

Solution 15-12. When it is apparent that a client is in need of professional services not offered in your clinic setting, a general referral for those services should be made.

Procedure for Making General Referrals for Psychological, Behavioral, Relational, Social, or Vocational Problems

A person who becomes so depressed by hearing loss that he or she does not go to work or out of the home for recreational or social activities may be suffering from clinical depression and should be referred for psychological counseling. Your report may state the referral in general terms, such as "Mr. Jones appears to be depressed over his hearing loss to the extent that the depression is interfering with his daily activities. He should be seen for psychological evaluation and counseling." Before making a specific referral to an outside agency for services, you must know the client's needs and what outside services are available to meet those needs. The client should acknowledge the need for and be willing to accept the services provided by the outside referral source.

Problem 15-13. Selection of a professional counselor to refer to for psychological, emotional, or interpersonal counseling.

Solution 15-13. Most practicum settings will have a list of referral sources for psychological counseling.

Procedure for Utilizing Outside Referrals for Psychological, Behavioral, or Interpersonal Problems

Counselors on the referral lists often are chosen because they have experience working with persons with hearing impairment and the services that they provide are consistent with the management goals of the practicum site.

In the area of interpersonal, emotional, and behavioral counseling, services may be offered by psychiatrists, psychologists, social workers, or marriage and family counselors. Psychiatrists are physicians with special training in relational, emotional, and behavioral disorders. As physicians, they diagnose emotional, behavioral, and personality disorders. They may prescribe drug treatment programs as a cure for emotional and behavioral disorders.

Psychologists, on the other hand, are not physicians. They hold advanced graduate and professional degrees like the Doctor of Philosophy (Ph.D.) and Psychology Doctorate (Psy. D.). Psychologists, like psychiatrists, diagnose emotional, behavioral, and personality disorders. Rather than prescribing drugs as therapy, psychologists rely on various counseling techniques to effect attitudinal, emotional, or behavioral change. Psychologists may be from one of two major schools of thought: behavioral or Freudian psychology. Behavioral psychologists use behavior modification techniques to change behaviors. Freudian psychologists probe the individual's past for significant events that may be brought into the individual's consciousness, and dealt with in such a way that the individual becomes emotionally or behaviorally healthy.

Social workers are professionals who identify governmental, community, educational and other resources for individuals in need of them. Many hospitals employ social workers to facilitate patient care. Social workers often are the case workers in county welfare and child protective services.

Marriage and family counselors are professionals who treat interpersonal or behavioral problems. These professionals examine the dynamics of interpersonal interactions and attempt to effect change with alternative coping strategies.

Hearing loss may aggravate existing interpersonal, emotional, and behavioral problems in individuals. Also, individuals with psychological, emotional, behavioral or interpersonal problems may acquire hearing loss. For clients who are not under treatment currently for interpersonal problems, referral to a marriage and family counselor is appropriate. For individuals with psychological, emotional, and behavioral problems, referral to a psychologist is appropriate. If the psychological, emotional, or behavioral problems result from a chemical imbalance in the individual, psychiatric referral is appropriate.

Problem 15-14. When should a client be referred to social and vocational services?

Solution 15-14. Referral for social or vocational services should be made when the client indicates a need for those services.

**Procedure for Utilizing Outside Referrals
for Social or Vocational Problems**

Hearing impairment can have social and vocational effects. In addition, persons who have social and vocational needs may become hearing impaired. Social and vocational services are available from a variety of sources. Some clinics that offer audiology services also employ social workers and vocational counselors. Most state and county governments administer programs that provide social and vocational services for those in need. A limited number of private vocational services are also available. In addition, many civic clubs, church groups, and religious organizations provide social and vocational assistance to those in need. All of these resources are important in meeting the needs of the community. You should become familiar with social and vocational services available in the area in which you will be doing your practicum.

Criteria for referral to these programs vary. Some programs provide a safe haven from abuse and neglect. Others provide assistance in combating alcohol and drug problems. Still others provide financial aid. There are programs that purchase diagnostic and rehabilitative services. Some programs, such as Medicaid, state Children's Services, and Vocational Rehabilitation departments purchase hearing aids for those who cannot afford them. Others provide job training. Whatever the client's vocational and social needs, there is a program to meet those needs. It is your responsibility to bring the need for referrals to the attention of your supervisor. In turn, you may be given the opportunity to make the referral and to follow up with the referring agency and the client.

Problem 15-15. A child between birth and 2 years of age has been diagnosed as profoundly hearing impaired and referred to you for communication training.

Solution 15-15. Counsel the parents regarding educational alternatives and the advantages of each.

Procedure for Counseling Parents Regarding Educational Alternatives for Children with Hearing impairment

Recommend that the child enroll in an appropriate educational program. If the child is visually oriented, unable to process auditory signals, or the goal of the parents is to develop communication as rapidly as possible, a manual approach can be considered. However, if the goal is to develop aural and oral communication as the primary mode of communication, the child should be enrolled in a program that emphasizes oral-aural communication. Cued speech uses hand signals to cue nonvisible sounds. Together with the visual cues of these sounds, tactile stimulation, or residual hearing, oral speech and language development can occur at a near normal rate. For speech and language to develop normally, interaction with peers is necessary. Enrolling the child in a day school program that emphasizes cued speech and parent training is a sensible option for the family who opts for oral-aural communication.

This chapter described audiologic management with techniques to modify psychological, social, and vocational variables associated with hearing impairment. Other chapters in this section introduced audiologic management related to medical and surgical treatment, amplification, and the modification of communicative behavior. Through the techniques offered in the chapters in Part IV , the needs of the client can be addressed. Addressing the needs of the client in a problem-solving format is the basis of successful client management.

References

Academy of Rehabilitative Audiology. (1992). General information. *Journal of the Academy of Rehabilitative Audiology, 25,* 1.

Alpiner, J. G., & McCarthy, P. A. (1993). *Rehabilitative audiology: Children and adults.* (2nd ed.). Baltimore: Williams & Wilkins.

American Auditory Society. (1992). AAS by laws. *AAS Bulletin, 17* (2), 108.

American National Standards Institute. Working Group ANSI 3.79-1990X. (1992). The ANSI Standard Method for calculation of the speech intelligibility index (Draft version ANSI 3.5-1990X).

American Speech-Language-Hearing Association. (1985). Guidelines for identification audiometry. *Asha, 27,* 49-52.

American Speech-Language-Hearing Association. (1989). Guidelines for audiologic screening of newborn infants who are at risk for hearing impairment. *Asha, 31* (3), 89-92.

American Speech-Language-Hearing Association. (1990a). Guidelines for screening for hearing impairments and middle ear disorders. *Asha, 32* (Suppl. 2), 17-24.

American Speech-Language-Hearing Association. (1990b). Position statement and guidelines. *Asha, 32* (4) (Suppl. 2).

American Speech-Language-Hearing Association. (1990c). Scope of practice, speech-language pathology and audiology. *Asha, 32* (4) (Suppl. 2), 1-2.

American Speech-Language-Hearing Association. (1990d). Standards for the certificates of clinical competence. *Asha, 32* (3), 111-112.

American Speech-Language-Hearing Association. (1991a). Position statement and guidelines. *Asha, 33* (3) (Suppl. 5).

American Speech-Language-Hearing Association. (1991b). Reports, tutorial and bibliography. *Asha, 33* (1) (Suppl. 3).

American Speech-Language-Hearing Association. (1992a). Audiologist respond to 1992 ASHA omnibus survey. *Audiology Update, 11* (1), 14-17.

American Speech-Language-Hearing Association. (1992b). Code of ethics. *Asha, 34* (3) (Suppl. 9), 1-2.

American Speech-Language-Hearing Association. (1992c). Guidelines, position statement, and report. *Asha, 34* (3) (Suppl. 7).

American Speech-Language-Hearing Association. (1993a). Guidelines for audiology services in the schools. *Asha, 35* (Suppl. 10), 24-32.

American Speech-Language-Hearing Association. (1993b). Preferred practice patterns for the professions of speech-language pathology and audiology. *Asha, 35* (3) (Suppl. 11).

American Speech-Language-Hearing Association. (1993c). Position statements and guidelines, and reports. *Asha, 35* (3) (Suppl. 10).

ASHA Clinical Certification Board. (1992). Implementation procedures for the standards for the certificate of clinical competence. *Asha, 34,* 72-79.

ASHA Committee on Infant Hearing. (1989). Audiologic screening of newborn infants who are at risk for hearing impairment. *Asha, 31,* 89-92.

ASHA Committee on Quality Assurance. (1989). AIDS/HIV: Implications for speech-language pathologists & audiologists. *Asha, 31,* 33.

ASHA Committee on Quality Assurance. (1990). Update. AIDS/HIV: Implications for speech-language pathologists & audiologists. *Asha, 32,* 46-48.

ASHA Committee on Supervision. (1985). Clinical supervision in speech-language pathology. *Asha, 27,* 57-60.

ASHA Council on Professional Standards in Speech-Language Pathology and Audiology. (1990). Standards for accreditation of educational programs. *Asha, 32,* 93-100.

ASHA Government Affairs Review. (1990). *Reauthorization of EHA discretionary programs.* Rockville, American Speech-Language-Hearing Association.

ASHA Joint Committee on Infant Hearing. (1982). Position statement. *Asha, 24,* (12), 1017-1018.

ASHA Membership and Certification Handbook-A. (1991). Rockville, MD: American Speech-Language-Hearing Association.

ASHA Professional Services Board. (1984). Organization and maintenance of records for clinical service delivery. *Asha, 26,* 39.

ASHA Subcommittee of the ASHA Committee on Communication Problems of the Aging. (1989). Draft for peer review: Guidelines for the identification of hearing impairment/handicap in adult elderly persons. *Asha, 31,* 59-63.

Benenson, A. S. (1990). *Control of communicable diseases in man* (15th ed.). Washington DC: American Public Health Association.

Bryne, D., & Dillon, H. (1986). The National Acoustics Laboratories' (NAL) new procedure for selecting gain and frequency response of a hearing aid. *Ear and Hearing, 7* (4), 257-265.

Burke, F. R. (1990). *Child abuse: Prevention and intervention.* Workshop presented at California State University, Fresno.

Davis, J. M., Elfenbein, J., Schum, R., & Bentler, R. A. (1986). Effects of mild and moderate hearing impairment on language, educational and psychosocial behavior of children. *Journal of Speech and Hearing Disorders, 51* (60), 53-62.

Decker, N. T. (Guest Ed.). (1992). Ottoacoustic emissions. *Seminars in Hearing, 13* (1), 1-104.

De Filippo, C. E., & Scott, B. L. (1978). A method for training and evaluating the reception of on-going speech. *Journal of the Acoustical Society of America, 63* (4), 1186-1192.

Dublinske, S., & Healey, W. C. (1978). P. L. 94-142: Questions and answers for the speech-language pathologist and audiologist. *Asha, 20,* 188-205.

Flower, R. (1984). *Delivery of speech-language pathology and audiology services.* Baltimore, Williams & Wilkins.

Garstecki, D. C. (1981). Auditory-visual training paradigm for hearing-impaired adults. *Journal Academy of Rehabilitative Audiology, 14,* 223-238.

Hall, J. W. (1992). *Handbook of auditory evoked responses.* Boston: Allyn and Bacon.

Hegde, M. N., & Davis, D. (1992). *Clinical methods and practicum in speech-language pathology.* San Diego: Singular Publishing Group.

Hood, L. J. (1992). Academy affairs: President's message. *Audiology Today, 4* (3), 2.

Hull, R. H. (1992). *Aural rehabilitation.* (2nd ed.). San Diego: Singular Publishing Group.

Joint Committee on Infant Hearing. (1991). 1990 position statement. *Asha, 33* (3) (Suppl. 5), 3-6.

Katz, J. (Ed.). (1985). *Handbook of clinical audiology* (3rd ed.). Baltimore: Williams & Wilkins.

Katz, J., Stecker, N. A., & Henderson, D. (1992). *Central auditory processing: A transdisciplinary view.* St. Louis: C. V. Mosby.

Katz, J., & Wilde, L. (1985). Auditory perceptual disorders in children. In J. Katz (Ed.), *Handbook of clinical audiology* (3rd ed., pp. 664-688). Baltimore: Williams & Wilkins.

Keith, R. W. (1981). Audiological and auditory-language tests of central auditory function. In R. W. Keith (Ed.), *Central auditory and language disorders in children.* (pp. 61-76). Houston: College-Hill Press.

Kryter, K. D. (1985). *The effects of noise on man.* New York: Academic Press.

Lamb, S. H., Owens, E., & Schubert, E. D. (1983). The revised form of the hearing performance inventory. *Ear and Hearing, 4* (3), 152-157.

Lynch, C. (1990). Characteristics of state licensure laws. *Asha, 32,* 47-55.

Lynn, G. E., & Gilroy, J. (1984). Detection and localization of central auditory disorders. In J. L. Northern (Ed.), *Hearing disorders* (2nd ed., pp. 179-192). Boston: Little, Brown.

Martin, F. N. (1991). *An introduction to audiology* (4th ed.). Englewood Cliffs, NJ: Prentice-Hall.

McMillan, M. O., & Willette, S. J. (1988). Aseptic technique: A procedure for preventing disease transmission in the practice environment. *Asha, 30,* 35-37.

Mecklenberg, D. J. (1990). Cochlear implants and rehabilitative practices. In R. E. Sandlin (Ed.), *Handbook of hearing aid amplification. Volume II: Clinical considerations and fitting practices* (pp. 179-202). Boston: College-Hill Press.

Meier, S. T., & Davis, S. R. (1993). *The elements of counseling* (2nd ed.). Pacific Grove, CA: Brooks/Cole.

Mueller, H. G., & Killion, M. (1990). An easy method for calculating the articulation index. *Hearing Journal, 43* (9), 14-17.

National Institutes of Health. (1993). Draft: Consensus development conference statement: Early identification of hearing impairment in infants and young children. Bethesda, Author.

Nerbonne, M. A., Smedley, T. C., Tannahill, J. C. Schow, R. L., & Flevaris-Phillips, C. (1989). Case studies: Adults/Elderly Adults. In R. L. Schow & M. A. Nerbonne (Eds.), *Introduction to aural rehabilitation* (2nd ed., pp. 541-573). Austin, TX: Pro-Ed.

Niswander, P. S. (1989). Listening checks on hearing instruments. *Hearing Instruments, 40* (4), 38-41.

Occupational Safety and Health Administration. (1983). Occupational noise exposure; hearing conservation admendment, Final Rule, *Federal Register, 48* (46), 9738-9785.

Quigley, S. P. (1968). *Some effects of hearing impairment upon school performance.* Springfield, IL: Division of Special Education Services, Department of Special Education Development and Education, State of Illinois.

Roberts, S. D., & Bouchard, K. R. (1989). Eastablishing rapport in rehabilitative audiology. *Journal Academy of Rehabilitative Audiology, 22,* 65-72.

Roberts, S. D., & Bryant, J. D. (1992). Establishing Counseling goals in rehabilitative audiology. *Journal Academy of Rehabilitative Audiology, 25,* 81-97.

Ross, M., & Giolas, T. G. (1978). Introduction. In M. Ross & T. G. Giolas (Eds.), *Auditory management of hearing impaired children* (pp. 1-13). Baltimore: University Park Press.

Sanders, D. A. (1993). *Management of hearing handicap: Infants to elderly* (3rd ed.). Englewood Cliffs, NJ: Prentice-Hall.

Sandlin, R. E. (Ed.). (1988). *Handbook of hearing aid amplification. Volume I: Theoretical and echnical considerations.* Boston: College-Hill Press.

Sandlin, R. E. (Ed.). (1990). *Handbook of hearing aid amplification. Volume II: Clinical considerations and fitting practices.* Boston: College-Hill Press.

Schow, R. L., & Nerbonne, M. A. (1989). *Introduction to aural rehabilitation.* (2nd ed.) Austin, TX: Pro-Ed.

Schow, R. L., & Nerbonne, M. A. (1992). Communication screening profile: Use with elderly clients. *Ear and Hearing, 3,* 135-147.

Turner, R. G. (1990). Recommended guidelines for infant hearing screening: analysis. *Asha, 32,* 57-61, 66.

Wall, L. G., Naples, G. M., Buhrer, K., & Capodanno, C. (1985). Audiological services within the school system. *Asha, 27,* 31-34.

Appendix A

Glossary of Medical Abbreviations and Symbols

Every profession has frequently used abbreviations, acronyms, and symbols. As you know, audiologists routinely use the abbreviations Hz (hertz) and dB (decibels), and the symbols X (left ear) and O (right eary) to record responses on audiograms. While working in medical settings, you may encounter many new abbreviations, acronyms, and symbols. Some of these are listed below.

ABI:	Acquired brain injury
a.c.:	Before meals
ACU:	Ambulatory Care Unit or Acute Care Unit
AL:	Allergy
A/O:	Alert and oriented
b.i.d.:	Twice daily
b.i.n.:	Twice nightly
c̄:	With
CA:	Cancer
CHI:	Closed head injury
CNS:	Central nervous system
CVA:	Cerebrovascular accident
DC (D/C):	Discontinue (Discharge)

Dx:	Diagnosis
EENT:	Eyes-ears-nose-throat
F.U.O.:	Fever of unknown origin
fx:	Fracture
h:	Hour
ICU:	Intensive Care Unit
LBW:	Low birth weight
NPO:	Nothing by mouth
O.D.:	Right eye
O.S.:	Left eye
O.T.:	Occupational therapist
O.U.:	Both eyes
p.o.:	By mouth
p.r.n.:	When necessary
P.T.:	Physical therapy
pt.:	Patient
q:	Every
Rx:	Prescription (Treatment)
s̄:	Without
stat:	Immediately
tpr:	Temperature-pulse-respiration
Tx:	Therapy (treatment)
♀:	Female
♂:	Male
↑:	Above (Increase)
↓:	Below (Decrease)
0:	Absent
∅:	None

Appendix B

Glossary of Educational Abbreviations and Acronyms

Following are some commonly used abbreviations and acronyms you may encounter in educational settings. There may be some variation across school sites, so check with your school to make sure you are using the correct abbreviations and acronyms.

ADA:	Average daily attendance
ADHD:	Attention deficit and Hyperactivity disorder
CH:	Communicatively handicapped
DD:	Developmentally disabled
DIS:	Designated instructional service
ED:	Emotionally disturbed
EDGAR:	Education Department General Administrative Regulations
EHA:	Education of the Handicapped Act (now known as IDEA)
ESL:	English as a second language
FAPE:	Free appropriate public education
FEP:	Fluent English proficient
HI:	Hearing-impaired

IDEA:	Individuals with Disabilities Education Act
IEP:	Individualized Education Program
IFSP:	Individualized Family Service Plan
LD:	Learning disability/learning disabled
LEP:	Limited English proficient
LES:	Limited English speaking
LH:	Learning handicapped
LRE:	Least restrictive environment
NES:	Non-English speaking
OCR:	Office for Civil Rights
OH:	Orthopedically handicapped
OSEP:	Office of Special Education Programs
PLP:	Present levels of performance
RS:	Resource specialist
SDC:	Special day class
SED:	Severely emotionally disturbed
SH:	Severely handicapped
SLH:	Speech-language-hearing specialist
SST:	Student study team

Appendix C

Code of Ethics
January 1, 1992
American Speech-Language-Hearing Association

Preamble

The preservation of the highest standards of integrity and ethical principles is vital to the responsible discharge of obligations in the professions of speech-language pathology and audiology. This Code of Ethics sets forth the fundamental principles and rules considered essential to this purpose.

Every individual who is (a) a member of the American Speech-Language-Hearing Association, whether certified or not, (b) a nonmember holding the Certificate of Clinical Competence from the Association, (c) an applicant for membership or certification, or (d) a Clinical Fellow seeking to fulfill standards for certification shall abide by this Code of Ethics.

Any action that violates the spirit and purpose of this Code shall be considered unethical. Failure to specify any particular responsibility or practice in this Code of Ethics shall not be construed as denial of the existence of such responsibilities or practices.

The fundamentals of ethical conduct are described by Principles of Ethics and by Rules of Ethics as they relate to responsibility to persons served, to the public, and to the professions of speech-language pathology and audiology.

Principles of Ethics, aspirational and inspirational in nature, form the underlying moral basis for the Code of Ethics. Individuals shall observe these principles as affirmative obligations under all conditions of professional activity.

Rules of Ethics are specific statements of minimally acceptable professional conduct or of prohibitions and are applicable to all individuals.

Principle of Ethics I

Individuals shall honor their responsibility to hold paramount the welfare of persons they serve professionally.

Rules of Ethics

A. Individuals shall provide all services competently.
B. Individuals shall use every resource, including referral when appropriate, to ensure that high-quality service is provided.
C. Individuals shall not discriminate in the delivery of services on the basis of race, sex, age, religion, national origin, sexual orientation, or handicapping condition.
D. Individuals shall fully inform the persons they serve of the nature and possible effects of services rendered and products dispensed.
E. Individuals shall evaluate the effectiveness of services rendered and of products dispensed and shall provide services or dispense products only when benefit can reasonably be expected.
F. Individuals shall not guarantee the results of any treatment or procedure, directly or by implication; however, they may make a reasonable statement of prognosis.
G. Individuals shall not evaluate or treat speech, language, or hearing disorders solely by correspondence.
H. Individuals shall maintain adequate records of professional services rendered and products dispensed and shall allow access to these records when appropriately authorized.

I. Individuals shall not reveal, without authorization, any professional or personal information about the person served professionally, unless required by law to do so, or unless doing so is necessary to protect the welfare of the person or the community.
J. Individuals shall not charge for services not rendered, nor shall they misrepresent,[1] in any fashion, services rendered or products dispensed.
K. Individuals shall use persons in research or as subjects of teaching demonstrations only with their informed consent.
L. Individuals shall withdraw from professional practice when substance abuse or an emotional or mental disability may adversely affect the quality of services they render.

Principle of Ethics II

Individuals shall honor their responsibility to achieve and maintain the highest level of professional competence.

Rules of Ethics

A. Individuals shall engage in the provision of clinical services only when they hold the appropriate Certificate of Clinical Competence or when they are in the certification process and are supervised by an individual who holds the appropriate Certificate of Clinical Competence.
B. Individuals shall engage in only those aspects of the professions that are within the scope
C. Individuals shall continue their professional development throughout their careers.
D. Individuals shall delegate the provision of clinical services only to persons who are certified or to persons in the education or certification process who are appropriately supervised. The provision of support services may be delegated to persons who are neither certified nor in the certification process only when a certificate holder provides appropriate supervision.
E. Individuals shall prohibit any of their professional staff from providing services that exceed the staff member's competence,

---

[1] For purposes of this Code of Ethics, misrepresentation includes any untrue statements or statements that are likely to mislead. Misrepresentation also includes the failure to state any information that is material and that ought, in fairness, to be considered.

considering the staff member's level of education, training, and experience.

F. Individuals shall ensure that all equipment used in the provision of services is in proper working order and is properly calibrated.

Principle of Ethics III

Individuals shall honor their responsibility to the public by promoting public understanding of the professions, by supporting the development of services designed to fulfill the unmet needs of the public, and by providing accurate information in all communications involving any aspect of the professions.

Rules of Ethics

A. Individuals shall not misrepresent their credentials, competence, education, training, or experience.

B. Individuals shall not participate in professional activities that constitute a conflict of interest.

C. Individuals shall not misrepresent diagnostic information, services rendered, or products dispensed or engage in any scheme or artifice to defraud in connection with obtaining payment or reimbursement for such services or products.

D. Individuals' statements to the public shall provide accurate information about the nature and management of communication disorders, about the professions, and about professional services.

E. Individuals' statements to the public — advertising, announcing, and marketing their professional services, reporting research results, and promoting products — shall adhere to prevailing professional standards and shall not contain misrepresentations.

Principles of Ethics IV

Individuals shall honor their responsibilities to the professions and their relationships with colleagues, students, and members of allied professions. Individuals shall uphold the dignity and autonomy of the professions, maintain harmonious interprofessional and intraprofessional relationships, and accept the professions' self imposed standards.

Rules of Ethics

A. Individuals shall prohibit anyone under their supervision from engaging in any practice that violates the Code of Ethics.
B. Individuals shall not engage in dishonesty, fraud, deceit, misrepresentation, or any form of conduct that adversely reflects on the professions or on the individual's fitness to serve persons professionally.
C. Individuals shall assign credit only to those who have contributed to a publication, presentation, or product. Credit shall be assigned in proportion to the contribution and only with the contributor's consent.
D. Individual's statements to colleagues about professional services, research results, and products shall adhere to prevailing professional standards and shall contain no misrepresentations.
E. Individuals shall not provide professional services without exercising independent professional judgment, regardless of referral source or prescription.
F. Individuals who have reason to believe that the Code of Ethics has been violated shall inform the Ethical Practice Board.
G. Individuals shall cooperate fully with the Ethical Practice Board in its investigation and adjudication of matters related to this Code of Ethics. (pp. 1-2)

Appendix D

Hearing Performance Inventory
Revised Form[1]
July, 1979

Instructions

We are interested in knowing how your hearing problem has affected your daily living. Below you will find a series of questions which describe a variety of everyday listening situations and ask you to judge how much difficulty you would have hearing in these situations.

Some of the questions ask you to judge how well you can understand what people are saying when their voices are loud enough. The term *understand* means hearing the words a person is saying clearly enough to be able to participate in the conversation. Other questions ask whether you can hear enough of a particular sound (doorbell, speech, etc.) to be aware of its presence. Other questions concern occupational, social or personal situations. Still others ask what you *do* when you miss something. Always assume you are interested in what is being said.

To answer each question, you are asked to check the phrase that best describes how often you experience the situation being described:

[1] Reprinted from Lamb, S. H., Owens, E., Schubert, E. D., & Giolas, T. G. *Hearing Performance Inventory — Revised,* with permission. (Available from Stanford H. Lamb, Ph.D., San Francisco State University.)

Practically always .... (or always)
Frequently .... (about three-quarters of the time)
About half the time
Occasionally .... (about a quarter of the time)
Almost never .... (or never)

For example, if you can understand what a person is saying on the telephone about 100% of the time, then you should check *practically always.* On the other hand, if you can understand almost nothing of what a person is saying on the telephone, then you should check *almost never.* If you can understand what a person is saying on the telephone about 50% of the time, then you should check *about half the time.*

Your answers to the questions should describe your present hearing ability as it is on the average rather than from a single instance.

If you wear a hearing aid in the situation described, answer the question accordingly.

Please check one, and only one, phrase for each question. You should check *Does not apply* only if you have not experienced a particular situation or one similar to it.

Questions that appear identical do differ in at least one important detail. Please read each question carefully before checking the appropriate phrase.

We know that people talk differently. Some mumble, others talk too fast, and others talk without moving their lips very much. Please answer the questions according to the way *most* people talk to you.

If the question does not specify whether the person speaking is male or female, answer according to which sex you have the most difficulty hearing.

Asterisks on the score sheet are for scoring purposes and should be ignored.

1. You are watching your favorite news program on television. Can you understand the news reporter (female) when her voice is loud enough for you?

2. You are reading in a room with music or noise in the background. Can you hear a person calling you from another room?

3. You are with a male friend or family member in a fairly quiet room. Can you understand him when his voice is loud enough for you and you can see his face?

4. Can you hear an airplane in the sky when others around you can hear it?

5. You are watching a drama or movie on television. Can you understand what is being said when the speaker's voice is loud enough for you and there is music in the background?

6. Can you understand what a woman is saying on the telephone when her voice is loud enough for you?

7. You are at a restaurant and you hear only a portion of something the waitress/waiter said. Do you repeat the portion when asking him/her for a repetition?

8. You are with a child (6 to 10 years old) in a fairly quiet room. Can you understand the child when his/her voice is loud enough for you and you can see his/her face?

9. You are the driver in an automobile with several friends or family members. One or more of the windows are open. Can you understand the passenger behind you when his/her voice is loud enough for you?

10. You are at a restaurant and there is background noise such as music or a crowd of people. Can you understand the waiter/waitress when his/her voice is loud enough for you and you can see his/her face?

11. You are talking with a close friend. When you miss something important that was said, do you immediately adjust your hearing aid to help you hear better?

12. You are with five or six strangers at a gathering of more than twenty people and there is background noise such as music or a crowd of people. One person talks at a time. When you are aware of the subject, can you understand what is being said when the speaker's voice is loud enough for you and you can see his/her face?

13. You are at a play or movie, or listening to a speech. When you miss something important that was said, do you ask the person with you?

14. You are with child (6 to 10 years old) and several people are talking nearby. Can you understand the child when his/her voice is loud enough for you and you can see his/her face?

15. You are playing cards, monopoly or some similar game with several people and there is background noise such as music or a crowd of people. Can you understand what a friend or family member is saying to you when his/her voice is loud enough for you and you can see his/her face?

16. Does your hearing problem discourage you from attending lectures?

17. You are talking with five or six friends. When you miss something that was said, do you ask the person talking to repeat it?

18. You are in an auditorium listening to a lecturer (female) who is using a microphone. Can you understand what she is saying when her voice is loud enough for you and you can see her face?

19. Can you hear water running in another room when others around you can hear it?

20. You are with a friend or family member and you hear only a portion of what was said. Do you repeat that portion when asking him/her for a repetition?

21. You are at a party or gathering of less than ten people and the room is fairly quiet. Can you understand what a friend or family member is saying to you when his/her voice is loud enough for you, but you can *not* see his/her face?

22. Does your hearing problem lower you self confidence?

23. You are in a fairly quiet room with five or six strangers. One person talks at a time. When you are aware of the subject, can you understand what is being siad when the speaker's voice is loud enough for you, but you can *not* see his/her face?

24. You are with five or six friends or family members at a gathering of more than twenty people and several people are talking near by. One person talks at a time and the subject of conversation changes from time to time. Can you understand what is being said when the speaker's voice is loud enough for you and you can see his/her face?

25. When an announcement is given over a public address system in a bus station or airport, is it *loud enough* for you to hear?

26. You are talking with a stranger. When you miss something important that was said, do you ask for it to be repeated?

27. You are talking with a friend or family member. When you miss something that was said, do you pretend you understood?

28. You are at a fairly quiet restaurant. Can you understand the waiter/waitress when his/her voice is loud enough for you and you can see his/her face?

29. You are seated with five or six strangers around a table or in a living room. Often two persons are talking at once and one person frequently interrupts another. When you miss something important that was said, do you pretend you understood?

30. You are playing cards, monopoly or some similar game and the room is fairly quiet. The subject of conversation changes from time to time. Can you understand what is being said when the speaker's voice is loud enough for you, but you can *not* see his/her face?

31. You are at a party or gathering of less than ten people and the room is fairly quiet. Can you understand what a friend or family member is saying to you when his/her voice is loud enough for you and you can see his/her face?

32. Does your hearing problem discourage you from going to concerts?

33. Do you find that children (6 to 10 years old) speak loudly enough for you?

34. When an announcement is given over a public address system in a bus station or airport, can you understand what is being said when the speaker's voice is loud enough for you?

35. You are seated with five or six strangers around a table or in a living room. Often two persons are talking at once and one person frequently interrupts another. Can you understand what is being said when the speaker's voice is loud enough for you and you can see his/her face?

36. You are seated with five or six friends around a table or in a living room. Often two persons are talking at once and one person frequently interrupts another. When you miss something that was said, do you ask the person talking to repeat it?

37. You are with a female stranger in a fairly quiet room. Can you understand her when her voice is loud enough for you and you can see her face?

38. You are with a stranger and there is background noise such as music or a crowd of people. Can you understand the person when his/her voice is loud enough for you, but you can *not* see his/her face?

39. Does your hearing problem tend to make you impatient?

40. You are talking with five or six strangers. When you miss something important that was said, do you let the person talking know—at least one time—that you have a hearing problem?

41. You are at a party or gathering of less than ten people and several people are talking near by. Can you understand what a friend or family member (female) is saying to you when her voice is loud enough for you and you can see her face?

42. Does your hearing problem discourage you from going to plays?

43. You are having dinner with five or six friends and you hear only a portion of what was said. Do you repeat that portion when asking the speaker for a repetition?

44. You are at a restaurant with a friend or family member and there is background noise such as music or a crowd of people. Can you understand the person when his/her voice is loud enough for you and you can see his/her face?

45. When you have difficulty understanding a person who speaks quite rapidly, do you ask him/her to speak more slowly?

46. You are talking to a woman sitting in a ticket or information booth and it is fairly noisy. She is giving directions or information. Can

you understand her when her voice is loud enough for you and you can see her face?

47. You are having dinner with five or six friends. When you miss something important that was said, do you ask the person talking to repeat it?

48. When others are listening to speech on the television or radio, is it loud enough for you?

49. Does your hearing problem discourage you from going to the movies?

50. You are riding in an automobile with several friends or family members. One or more of the windows are open and you are sitting in the front seat. Can you understand the driver when his/her voice is loud enough for you and you can see his/her face?

51. You are at home watching television or listening to the radio. Can you hear the doorbell ring when it is located in the same room?

52. You are in a fairly quiet room talking with five or six strangers. One person talks at a time and the subject of conversation changes from time to time. Can you understand what is being said when the speaker's voice is loud enough for you and you can see his/her face?

53. You are seated with five or six friends or family members around a table or in a living room. Often two persons are talking at once and one person frequently interrupts another. When you miss something important that was said, do you remind the person talking, at least once, that you have a hearing problem?

54. You are attending a stage play. Can you understand what the actors/actresses are saying when their voices are loud enough for you and you can see their faces?

55. You are with a friend or family member in a fairly quiet room. Can you understand him/her when his/her voice is loud enough for you, but you can *not* see his/her face?

56. A person is talking to you from a distance of no more than six feet. There is music or noise in the background. Would you be aware that he/she is talking if you did not see his/her face?

57. You are having dinner with five or six friends or family members at home and there is background noise such as music or a crowd of people. Can you understand what is being said when the speaker's voice is loud enough for you, but you can *not* see his/her face?

58. When you have difficulty understanding a person with a pipe, toothpick or similar object in his/her mouth, do you ask him/her to remove the object?

59. You are the driver in an automobile with several friends or family members. The windows are closed. Can you understand the passenger behind you when his/her voice is loud enough for you?

60. When you have difficulty understanding a person because he is holding his hand in front of his mouth, do you ask him to lower his hand?

61. You are at a party or gathering of more than twenty people and there is background noise such as music or a crowd of people. Can you understand what a stranger is saying to you when his/her voice is loud enough for you and you can see his/her face?

62. Do you feel that others cannot understand what it is to have a hearing problem?

63. You are at a movie. Can you understand what the actors/actresses are saying when their voices are loud enough for you and you can see their faces?

64. You are talking with five or six strangers. When you miss something important that was said, do you ask the person talking to repeat it?

65. You are at a party or gathering of more than twenty people and several people are talking near by. Can you understand what a friend or family member (male) is saying to you when his voice is loud enough for you and you can see his face?

66. You are in a fairly quiet room. Can you carry on a conversation with a man in another room if his voice is loud enough for you?

67. You are with a male friend or family member and several people are talking near by. Can you understand him when his voice is loud enough for you and you can see his face?

68. You are with five or six friends or family members. One person talks at a time. When you miss something important that was said, do you pretend you understood?

69. You are watching a drama or movie on television. Can you understand what is being said when the speaker's voice is loud enough for you and there is no music in the background?

70. You are with five or six friends or family members and there is background noise such as music or a crowd of people. One person talks at a time. When you are aware of the subject, can you understand what is being said when the speaker's voice is loud enough for you, but you can *not* see his/her face?

71. You are at a lecture. If you have difficulty hearing what is being said, do you move to a place where you can hear better?

72. Does your hearing problem tend to make you feel nervous or tense?

73. You are with a female stranger and there is background noise such as traffic, music, or a crowd of people. Can you understand her when her voice is loud enough for you and you can see her face?

74. You are in a quiet place and the person seated on the side of your better ear whispers to you. Can you hear the whisper?

75. You are at a small social gathering. If you have difficulty hearing what is being said, do you move to a place where you can hear better?

Occupational Items

76. You are with a male co-worker at work in a fairly quiet room. Can you understand him when his voice is loud enough for you and you can see his face?

77. You are with five or six co-workers at work. One person talks at a time. When you miss something important that was said, do you pretend you understand?

78. Does your hearing problem interfere with helping or instructing others on the job?

79. You are with a female co-worker at work and there is background noise such as traffic, music, or a crowd of people. Can you understand her when her voice is loud enough for you and you can see her face?

80. You are with a co-worker at work and you hear only a portion of what was said. Do you repeat that portion when asking the speaker for a repetition?

81. You are talking with a co-worker at work. When you miss something important that was said, do you ask for it to be repeated?

82. You are talking with your employer (foreman, supervisor, etc.) and several people are talking near by. Can you understand him/her when his/her voice is loud enough for you and you can see his/her face?

83. You are with a female co-worker at work in a fairly quiet room. Can you understand her when her voice is loud enough for you and you can see her face?

84. You are talking with a co-worker or employer. When you miss something important that was said, do you remind him/her that you have a hearing problem?

85. You are in a fairly quiet room at work with five or six co-workers. One person talks at a time and the subject of conversation changes from time to time. Can you understand what is being said when the speaker's voice is loud enough for you and you can see his/her face?

86. Does your hearing problem interfere with learning the duties of a new job easily?

87. You are seated with five or six co-workers around a table at work. Often two persons are talking at once and one person frequently interrupts another. Can you understand what is being said when the speaker's voice is loud enough for you and you can see his/her face?

88. You are talking with a co-worker at work. When you miss something important that was said, do you pretent you understood?

89. You are with a male co-worker at work and there is background noise such as traffic, music, or a crowd of people. Can you understand him when his voice is loud enough for you and you can see his face?

90. You are talking with a co-worker at work. When you miss something that was said, do you immediately adjust your hearing aid to help you hear better?

Sections

Understanding Speech
  With Visual Cues 1, 3, 5, 8, 10, 12, 14, 15, 18, 24, 28, 31, 35, 37, 41, 44, 46, 50, 52, 54, 61, 63, 65, 67, 69, 73
  With No Visual Cues 6, 9, 21, 23, 30, 34, 38, 55, 57, 59, 66, 70
Intensity 2, 4, 19, 25, 33, 48, 51, 56, 74
Response to Auditory Failure 7, 11, 13, 17, 20, 26, 27, 29, 36, 40, 43, 45, 47, 53, 58, 60, 64, 68, 71, 75
Personal 16, 22, 32, 39, 42, 49, 62, 72
Social 9, 12, 15, 17, 21, 23, 24, 29, 30, 31, 35, 36, 40, 41, 43, 47, 50, 52, 53, 57, 59, 61, 64, 65, 68, 70, 75
Occupational
  Understanding Speech With Visual Cues 76, 79, 82, 83, 85, 87, 89
  Response to Auditory Failure 77, 80, 81, 84, 88, 90
  Personal 78, 86

Categories and Subcategories

Social items are underlined, occupational items parenthesized

Understanding Speech (with Visual Cues)
  Talker
    Male 3, 67, 65, (76, 89)

HEARING PERFORMANCE INVENTORY (REVISED FORM)

79-334P

NAME ______ AGE ______ DATE ______

ADDRESS ______ PHONE ______

TEST LOCATION ______ SEX ______ MARITAL STATUS ______

EMPLOYED ______ EDUCATION ______ HEARING AID WEARER: Yes ☐ No ☐

PRIOR AURAL REHABILITATION COURSE EXPERIENCE? ______ IF YES, WHEN? ______

Item	Practically Always	Frequently	About Half The Time	Occasionally	Almost Never	Does Not Apply
1.	☐	☐	☐	☐	☐	☐
2.	☐	☐	☐	☐	☐	☐
3.	☐	☐	☐	☐	☐	☐
4.	☐	☐	☐	☐	☐	☐
5.	☐	☐	☐	☐	☐	☐
6.	☐	☐	☐	☐	☐	☐
7.	☐	☐	☐	☐	☐	☐
8.	☐	☐	☐	☐	☐	☐
9.	☐	☐	☐	☐	☐	☐
10.	☐	☐	☐	☐	☐	☐
11.	☐	☐	☐	☐	☐	☐
12.	☐	☐	☐	☐	☐	☐
13.	☐	☐	☐	☐	☐	☐
14.	☐	☐	☐	☐	☐	☐
15.	☐	☐	☐	☐	☐	☐
* 16.	☐	☐	☐	☐	☐	☐
17.	☐	☐	☐	☐	☐	☐
18.	☐	☐	☐	☐	☐	☐
19.	☐	☐	☐	☐	☐	☐
20.	☐	☐	☐	☐	☐	☐
21.	☐	☐	☐	☐	☐	☐
* 22.	☐	☐	☐	☐	☐	☐
23.	☐	☐	☐	☐	☐	☐
24.	☐	☐	☐	☐	☐	☐
25.	☐	☐	☐	☐	☐	☐
26.	☐	☐	☐	☐	☐	☐
* 27.	☐	☐	☐	☐	☐	☐
28.	☐	☐	☐	☐	☐	☐
* 29.	☐	☐	☐	☐	☐	☐
30.	☐	☐	☐	☐	☐	☐
31.	☐	☐	☐	☐	☐	☐
* 32.	☐	☐	☐	☐	☐	☐
33.	☐	☐	☐	☐	☐	☐
34.	☐	☐	☐	☐	☐	☐
35.	☐	☐	☐	☐	☐	☐
36.	☐	☐	☐	☐	☐	☐
37.	☐	☐	☐	☐	☐	☐
38.	☐	☐	☐	☐	☐	☐
* 39.	☐	☐	☐	☐	☐	☐
40.	☐	☐	☐	☐	☐	☐
41.	☐	☐	☐	☐	☐	☐
* 42.	☐	☐	☐	☐	☐	☐
43.	☐	☐	☐	☐	☐	☐
44.	☐	☐	☐	☐	☐	☐
45.	☐	☐	☐	☐	☐	☐

Item	Practically Always	Frequently	About Half The Time	Occasionally	Almost Never	Does Not Apply
46.	☐	☐	☐	☐	☐	☐
47.	☐	☐	☐	☐	☐	☐
48.	☐	☐	☐	☐	☐	☐
* 49.	☐	☐	☐	☐	☐	☐
50.	☐	☐	☐	☐	☐	☐
51.	☐	☐	☐	☐	☐	☐
52.	☐	☐	☐	☐	☐	☐
53.	☐	☐	☐	☐	☐	☐
54.	☐	☐	☐	☐	☐	☐
55.	☐	☐	☐	☐	☐	☐
56.	☐	☐	☐	☐	☐	☐
57.	☐	☐	☐	☐	☐	☐
58.	☐	☐	☐	☐	☐	☐
59.	☐	☐	☐	☐	☐	☐
60.	☐	☐	☐	☐	☐	☐
61.	☐	☐	☐	☐	☐	☐
* 62.	☐	☐	☐	☐	☐	☐
63.	☐	☐	☐	☐	☐	☐
64.	☐	☐	☐	☐	☐	☐
65.	☐	☐	☐	☐	☐	☐
66.	☐	☐	☐	☐	☐	☐
67.	☐	☐	☐	☐	☐	☐
* 68.	☐	☐	☐	☐	☐	☐
69.	☐	☐	☐	☐	☐	☐
70.	☐	☐	☐	☐	☐	☐
71.	☐	☐	☐	☐	☐	☐
* 72.	☐	☐	☐	☐	☐	☐
73.	☐	☐	☐	☐	☐	☐
74.	☐	☐	☐	☐	☐	☐
75.	☐	☐	☐	☐	☐	☐
76.	☐	☐	☐	☐	☐	☐
* 77.	☐	☐	☐	☐	☐	☐
* 78.	☐	☐	☐	☐	☐	☐
79.	☐	☐	☐	☐	☐	☐
80.	☐	☐	☐	☐	☐	☐
81.	☐	☐	☐	☐	☐	☐
82.	☐	☐	☐	☐	☐	☐
83.	☐	☐	☐	☐	☐	☐
84.	☐	☐	☐	☐	☐	☐
85.	☐	☐	☐	☐	☐	☐
* 86.	☐	☐	☐	☐	☐	☐
87.	☐	☐	☐	☐	☐	☐
* 88.	☐	☐	☐	☐	☐	☐
89.	☐	☐	☐	☐	☐	☐
90.	☐	☐	☐	☐	☐	☐

* Items to be reversed before scoring.

Understanding Speech (with Visual Cues) *(continued)*
  Female 37, 1, 18, 73, *41,* 46, (83, 79)
  Child 8, 14
  Friend/family member 3, *31,* 67, 44, *41, 65, 15*
  Stranger 37, 73, *61*
  Co-worker (83, 76, 79, 89)
  Employer (82)
  Waiter/waitress 28, 10
Communicative Situation
  One-to-one 3, 37, 8, *31,* 67, 73, 14, 44, *41, 65, 61, 15,* (83, 76, 79, 89, 82)
    Alone 3, 37, 8, 67, 73, 14, 44, (83, 76, 79, 89, 82)
    In group < 10 *31, 41*
    In group > 20 *65, 61*
    In group playing
      cards, etc. *15*
  Group Conversation *52, 12, 24, 35, 50,* (85, 87)
    5 or 6 friends/family members within group < 20 *24*
    5 or 6 strangers *52, 35*
      within group < 20 *12*
    5 or 6 co-workers (85, 87)
    Several friends in automobile *50*
    One talker at a time
      Listener aware of subject *12*
      Subject changes *52, 24,* (85)
    Talkers interrupting *35,* (87)
Communication System
  Public address in auditorium 18
  Television
    News 1
    Drama or Movie 69, 5
  Movie 63
  Stage play 54
Noise Environment
  Fairly quiet 3, 37, 8, 28, *31, 52,* 69 (83, 76, 85)
  Music, etc. 5, 73, 10, 44, *61, 15, 12, 50,* 46, (79, 89)
  People talking nearby 67, 14, *41, 65, 24,* (82)
Miscellaneous
  Restaurant 28, 10, 44
  Ticket-information booth 46
Understanding Speech (No Visual Cues)
  Talker
    Male 66

Female 6
Friend/family member 55, *21*
Stranger 38
Communicative Situation
    One-to-one 66, 5, 38, 21
        Alone 55, 38
        Other room 66
        In group *21*
    Group Conversation *59, 9, 70, 23, 57, 30*
        5 or 6 friends/family members *70, 57*
        5 or 6 strangers *23*
        Automobile *59, 9*
        Games *30*
        One talker at a time
            Listener aware of subject *70, 23*
            Subject changes *30*
Communication System
    Telephone 6
    Public address, bus station 34
Noise Environment
    Fairly quiet 66, *59*, 55, *21, 23, 30*
    Music, etc. *9*, 38, *70, 57*
Intensity
Talker
    Child 33
    Communicative Situation (One-to-one)
    Other room 2
    Six feet away 56
    Whisper 74
    Communication System
    Public address, bus station, or airport 25
    Radio or TV 48
Non-speech
    Doorbell (same room) 51
    Airplane 4
    Water running 19
Noise Environment
    Quiet 74
    Music, etc. 2, 51, 56
Response to Auditory Failure
Talker
    Friend/family member 11, 27, 20
    Stranger 26

Appendix E

Self-Assessment of Communication

significant other assessment of communication (soac)

Name _____

Form filled out with reference to _____ (client/patient)

Informant's relationship to client/patient _____ (wife, son, friend, etc.)

Date _____

One of the following 5 descriptions should be assigned to each of the statements below. Circle a number from 1 to 5 next to each statement (Do not answer with yes or no).

1) Almost Never (or never)	2) Occasionally (about ¼ of the time)	3) About Half of the Time	4) Frequently (about ¾ of the time)	5) Practically always (or always)

Various Communication Situations	Circle number below
1. Does he/she experience communication difficulties in situations when speaking with one other person? (For example, at home, at work, in a social situation, with a waitress, a store clerk, with a spouse, boss, etc.)	1 2 3 4 5
2. Does he/she experience communication difficulties in situations when conversing with a small group of several persons? (For example, with friends or family, co-workers, in meetings or casual conversations, over dinner or while playing cards, etc.)	1 2 3 4 5
3. Does he/she experience communication difficulties while listening to a large group? (For example, at church or in a civic meeting, in a fraternal or women's club, at an educational lecture, etc.)	1 2 3 4 5

Continued

Source: From R. L. Schow and M. A. Nerbonne, *Introduction to aural rehabilitation.* © 1989 by Allyn & Bacon. Reprinted with permission.

Various Communication Situations (Continued)	Circle number below

4. Does he/she experience communication difficulties while participating in various types of entertainment? (For example, movies, TV, radio, plays, night clubs, musical entertainment, etc.)   1 2 3 4 5

5. Does he/she experience communication difficulties when you are in an unfavorable listening environment? (For example, at a noisy party, where there is background music, when riding in an auto or bus, when someone whispers or talks from across the room, etc.)   1 2 3 4 5

6. Does he/she experience communication difficulties when using or listening to various communication devices? (For example, telephone, telephone ring, doorbell, public address system, warning signals, alarms, etc.)   1 2 3 4 5

Feelings about Communication

7. Do you feel that any difficulty with his/her hearing limits or hampers his/her personal or social life?   1 2 3 4 5

8. Does any problem or difficulty with his/her hearing upset you?   1 2 3 4 5

Other People

9. Do others suggest that he/she has a hearing problem?   1 2 3 4 5

10. Do others leave him/her out of conversations or become annoyed because of his/her hearing?   1 2 3 4 5

Raw Score ___ × 2 = ___ − 20 = ___ × 1.25 ___ %

Appendix F

Fresno Auditory Feature Identification Test (FAFIT)

FORM I

(Grave/Acute)

1. fɑ fɑ
2. bɑ dɑ
3. sɑ fɑ
4. vɑ vɑ
5. fɑ sɑ
6. dɑ bɑ
7. vɑ zɑ
8. fɑ fɑ
9. sɑ sɑ
10. zɑ vɑ

(Compact/Diffuse)

11. ʒɑ zɑ
12. tɑ tɑ
13. zɑ ʒɑ
14. dɑ gɑ
15. θɑ θɑ
16. tɑ kɑ
17. ʃɑ ʃɑ
18. gɑ gɑ
19. sɑ ʃɑ
20. kɑ tɑ

(Tense/Lax)

21. vɑ vɑ
22. fɑ vɑ
23. dɑ dɑ
24. kɑ gɑ
25. θɑ ðɑ
26. dɑ tɑ
27. fɑ fɑ
28. ðɑ θɑ
29. bɑ bɑ
30. sɑ zɑ

(Strident/Mellow)

31. ðɑ ðɑ
32. θɑ sɑ
33. tʃɑ tʃɑ
34. sɑ θɑ
35. tʃɑ kɑ
36. ðɑ zɑ
37. d ʒɑ gɑ
38. θɑ θɑ
39. kɑ tʃɑ
40. d ʒɑ d ʒɑ

(Continuant/Interrupted)

41. bɑ vɑ
42. ðɑ ðɑ
43. vɑ bɑ
44. sɑ tɑ
45. tʃɑ tʃɑ
46. ðɑ dɑ
47. tɑ tɑ
48. dɑ ðɑ
49. tɑ sɑ
50. dɑ dɑ

333

FRESNO AUDITORY FEATURE IDENTIFICATION TEST (FAFIT)

RESPONSE FORM

Name _____

Date _____   Score _____

Form _____

Listening Conditions _____

Instructions: You will hear pairs of nonsense syllables. If the two members of each pair sound the same, mark S. If the two members of each pair sound different, mark D. If you are not sure, please guess. It is important that you mark either the S or the D for each item.

Practice set

1. S D			3. S D	
2. S D			4. S D	

1. S D	11. S D	21. S D	31. S D	41. S D
2. S D	12. S D	22. S D	32. S D	42. S D
3. S D	13. S D	23. S D	33. S D	43. S D
4. S D	14. S D	24. S D	34. S D	44. S D
5. S D	15. S D	25. S D	35. S D	45. S D
6. S D	16. S D	26. S D	36. S D	46. S D
7. S D	17. S D	27. S D	37. S D	47. S D
8. S D	18. S D	28. S D	38. S D	48. S D
9. S D	19. S D	29. S D	39. S D	49. S D
10. S D	20. S D	30. S D	40. S D	50. S D

334

Appendix G

A Signal Detection Method of Scoring

You may wish to obtain a measure of speech discrimination utilizing the FAFIT materials. When doing so, it is recommended that a detectibility index be calculated because the two-interval forced-choice response method of the test places chance at 50%. Therefore, a section on calculating the detectibility index is included in the first section of this appendix. The second section of the appendix shows how to calculate listener criterion. Both sections give examples of calculating and interpreting hypothetical scores.

Detectability Index (d')

There is a disadvantage to scoring the same-different response format by a percent correct method. Chance performance on each item would be 50%. The reduced range of scores (50-100%) may obscure significant differences in detectibility. Signal detection analysis scoring does not have this disadvantage. The formula for d' is:

$$d' = \text{ABS Hit Rate (HR)} - \text{ABS False Alarm Rate (FAR)}$$

where
ABS is the abcissa value of the standardized normal distribution for the proportion obtained. Abcissa values are obtained from a table of abcissa and ordinate values. Larry Hochhaus published such a table for the calculation of d' and β in the *Psychological Bulletin* (1972, Vol. 77, No. 5, pp. 375-376).

HR is the number of different item identified as different divided by the total number of different items.

FAR is the number of same items identified as different divided by the total number of same items.

An example of calculating d' follows:
If an individual identifies 25 of the 30 different items as different and 2 of the 20 items that are the same as different, the formula would contain the following values.

$$d' = ABS\ 25/30 - ABS\ 2/20$$

which reduces to ABS .83 - ABS .10 = .95417 - (- 1.28155) = 2.236 standard deviations above chance.
This score in percent correct would be 50 - 7 = 43 × 2 = 86%. Notice that pure guessing produces a d' of 0%.

$$d' = ABS\ 15/30 - ABS\ 10/20$$

which reduces to ABS .5 - ABS .5 = .000 - .000 = 0 difference with pure guessing behavior. This score in percent correct would be 50 - 25 = 25 × 2 = 50%. Notice that a very different score is produced by 6 hits and 1 false alarm, whereas the traditional percent correct score yields the same 50% score. Six different signals correctly identified and 19 same responses correctly identified totals 25 correct responses. Twenty-five times 2 is 50%.

$$d' = ABS\ 6/30 - ABS\ 1/20 = ABS\ .2 - ABS\ .05 = -.84162 - (- 1.6485) = .803$$

standard deviations above chance. The latter score represents better signal detection than the d' of 0. In percent correct there is no difference between the scores.

A Criterion Index

In addition to a detectibility index, signal detection scoring provides a measure of listener criterion (β). The formula for β is

$$\beta = \text{ORD HR/ORD FAR}$$

Where **ORD** is the ordinate value of the standardized normal distribution for the obtained proportions.
An example of calculating β follows:

If an individual identifies 25 of the 30 different items as different and 2 of the 20 same items as different the equation would be:

$$\beta = \frac{\text{ORD } 25/30}{\text{ORD } 10/20} \text{ which reduces to } \frac{\text{ORD } .83}{\text{ORD } .10} = \frac{.25305\ 35384}{.17549\ 83319} = .1442$$

Notice that pure guessing that produces a d' = 0 theoretically can produce a β = 1.0 if the criterion is based on a statistically perfect priori probability:

$$\beta = \frac{\text{ORD } 15/30}{\text{ORD } 10/20} = \text{ORD } .5/ \text{ ORD } .5 = .000/.000 = 1.0$$

Beta is independent of d'. A low d' or a high d' may produce a β of 1.0 if criterion. A β of 1.0 is the criterion at which most effective communicators function. A β score different than 1.0 may result from a conservative (less willing to guess) criterion or from a liberal (too willing to guess) criterion. Conservative criteria will be above 1.0, and liberal criteria will be lower than 1.0. Three examples will illustrate the calculating of β that result from conservative criteria. A fourth example is a β that resulted from a person with a too liberal criterion.

$$\beta = \frac{\text{ORD } 25/30}{\text{ORD } 1/20} = \text{ORD } .83/\text{ORD } .05 = \frac{.25305\ 35384}{.10313\ 56404} = 2.454$$

$$\beta = \frac{\text{ORD } 15/30}{\text{ORD } 1/20} = \text{ORD } .5/\text{ORD } .05 = \frac{.39894\ 22804}{.10313\ 56404} = 3.8681321$$

$$\beta = \frac{\text{ORD } 25/30}{\text{ORD } 0/20} = \text{ORD } .5/\text{ORD } .01 = \frac{.39894\ 22804}{.02665\ 21422} = 14.969$$

$$\beta = \frac{\text{ORD } 3/30}{\text{ORD } 5/20} = \text{ORD } .99/\text{ORD } .25 = \frac{.02665\ 21422}{.31777\ 65727} = .084$$

The more a person's β differs from 1.0, the less appropriate his or her criterion is for responding in communication.

Appendix H

Hearing Aid Evaluation

Hearing Aid Evaluation

Name _____   Date _____

	Right Ear								Left Ear					
250	500	1000	2000	3000	4000	6000		250	500	1000	2000	3000	4000	6000

___ ___ ___ ___ ___ ___ ___ | ___ ___ ___ ___ ___ ___ ___
(Threshold HL)   (Threshold HL)

Multiply threshold values by .5 above.

___ ___ ___ ___ ___ ___ | ___ ___ ___ ___ ___ ___
(Threshold SPL x multiplier)   (Threshold SPL x multiplier)

If available add the canal response to the threshold value x multiplier.

___ ___ ___ ___ ___ ___ | ___ ___ ___ ___ ___ ___
(Canal Response SPL)   (Canal Response SPL)

If the canal response is obtained, subtract Kemar values to obtain the hearing aid gain.

0   0   0   12   17   14 | 0   0   0   12   17   14

Add Reserve gain.

0   0   10   10   10   10 | 0   0   10   10   10   10

___ ___ ___ ___ ___ | ___ ___ ___ ___ ___
(2CC coupler full-on gain SPL)   (2CC coupler full-on gain SPL)

Maximum Power Output

___ ___ ___ ___ | ___ ___ ___ ___
(Gain + 65 dB SPL)   (Gain + 65 dB SPL)

340

	Right Ear							Left Ear						
250	500	1000	2000	3000	4000	6000		250	500	1000	2000	3000	4000	6000

___	___	___	___	___	___	___		___	___	___	___	___	___	___

(Uncomfortable Loudness HL)   (Uncomfortable Loudness HL)

20	6.0	2.0	4.0	5.0	5.0	11		20	6.0	2.0	4.0	5.0	5.0	11

(SPL Correction)   (SPL Correction)

___	___	___	___	___	___	___		___	___	___	___	___	___	___

(Uncomfortable Loudness SPL)   (Uncomfortable Loudness SPL)

Right Ear   Left Ear

_____   _____

(Most Comfortable Loudness Level for continuous speech in HL)

20   20
(SPL Correction)   (SPL Correction)

_____   _____

(Most Comfortable Loudness Level for continuous speech in SPL)

Automatic Volume Control

2 cc coupler full on gain + 65 dB SPL average input level of normal conversational speech - Threshold of Discomfort.

	Right Ear							Left Ear						
250	500	1000	2000	3000	4000	6000		250	500	1000	2000	3000	4000	6000

___	___	___	___	___	___	___		___	___	___	___	___	___	___

If positive number, automatic volume control is required.

To set the kneepoint of a compression-type instrument, subtract the largest value above from the lowest Threshold of Discomfort value.

_____   _____

Appendix I

Battery Life Chart

BATTERY LIFE CHART

Starkey

Battery Drain Current (ma) Per ANSI S3.22 1976	675								13						312								230		10A	
	MERC 235 mAh Hrs	Days	MERC 265 mAh Hrs	Days	ZINC AIR 520 mAh Hrs	Days	ZINC AIR 540 mAh Hrs	Days	MERC 95 mAh Hrs	Days	ZINC AIR 210 mAh Hrs	Days	ZINC AIR 230 mAh Hrs	Days	MERC 45 mAh Hrs	Days	MERC 55 mAh Hrs	Days	ZINC AIR 100 mAh Hrs	Days	ZINC AIR 110 mAh Hrs	Days	ZINC AIR 50 mAh Hrs	Days	ZINC AIR 60 mAh Hrs	Days
.2 ma	1175	73	1325	83	2600	163	2700	169	475	30	1050	66	1150	72	225	14	275	17	500	31	550	34	250	16	300	19
.3 ma	783	49	883	55	1733	108	1800	113	317	20	700	44	767	48	150	9	183	12	333	21	367	22	167	10	200	13
.4 ma	588	37	663	41	1300	81	1350	84	238	15	525	33	575	36	113	7	138	9	250	16	275	17	125	8	150	9
.5 ma	470	29	530	33	1040	65	1080	68	190	12	420	26	460	29	90	6	110	7	200	13	220	14	100	6	120	8
.6 ma	392	25	442	28	867	54	900	56	158	10	350	22	383	24	75	5	92	6	167	10	183	12	83	5	100	6
.7 ma	336	21	379	24	743	46	771	48	136	9	300	19	329	21	64	4	79	5	143	9	157	10	71	5	86	5
.8 ma	294	18	331	21	650	41	675	42	119	7	263	16	288	18	56	4	69	4	125	8	138	9	63	4	75	5
.9 ma	261	16	294	18	578	36	600	38	106	7	233	15	256	16	50	3	61	4	111	7	122	8	56	4	67	4
1.0 ma	235	15	265	17	520	33	540	34	95	6	210	13	230	14	45	3	55	3	100	6	110	7	50	3	60	4
1.2 ma	196	12	221	14	433	27	450	28	79	5	175	11	192	12	38	2	46	3	83	5	92	6	42	3	50	3
1.4 ma	168	11	189	12	371	23	386	24	68	4	150	9	164	10	32	2	39	3	71	5	79	5	36	2	43	3
1.6 ma	146	9	166	10	325	20	338	21	59	4	131	8	144	9	28	2	34	2	63	4	69	4	31	2	38	2
1.8 ma	131	8	147	9	289	18	300	19	53	3	117	7	128	8	25	2	31	2	56	4	61	4	28	2	33	2

$$\text{Battery Life (hours)} = \frac{\text{Battery mAh Rating}}{\text{Current Drain}}$$
$$\div \text{ Daily Use (hrs) } 16 = \text{Battery Life (days)}$$

- Battery life may vary with age of batteries (freshness)
- Battery life may vary with sound environment (push-pull circuits)
- All measurements are approximate

Battery life chart reprinted with permission of Starkey Laboratories, Inc.

Index